Josep de Haro Licer

From Taste to Disgust

Josep de Haro Licer

From Taste to Disgust

New vision of the perception of the sense of taste

ScienciaScripts

Imprint

Cover image: www.ingimage.com

This book is a translation from the original published under ISBN 978-613-9-40507-7.

Publisher:
Sciencia Scripts
is a trademark of
Dodo Books Indian Ocean Ltd. and OmniScriptum S.R.L publishing group

120 High Road, East Finchley, London, N2 9ED, United Kingdom
Str. Armeneasca 28/1, office 1, Chisinau MD-2012, Republic of Moldova, Europe
Printed at: see last page
ISBN: 978-620-7-96876-3

INDEX

1-Introduction

What does it mean to talk about taste? How does dislike form part of taste? These are the questions we are going to link together. To do so, the first thing we have to take into account is something that someone like Albert Einstein already asked himself and that Greek philosophers also asked themselves before:

What knowledge can thought acquire if it is independent of what the senses inform it?

This question means that we have to enter the realm of perception. And what does this realm tell us? Well, that we need senses. That they are our first level in the construction of perception.

Our perception depends on the modeling of the senses that is carried out by means of four factors: The **"phylogenic"** ones, which are those that govern the evolution-adaptation of the animal world until our species appears. The **"ontogenetic"** factors that condition sensoriality during gestation, via the genetic load of the progenitors, and the maternal and environmental influences, a phase in which the senses already begin to activate (the fetus sees, hears, smells, touches and tastes), capturing the external stimuli that the mother captures and the experiential stimuli that the mother experiences (emotions, feelings). The third group of factors, the **"sociogenic"** ones, are those that appear in a massive way when the fetus is already on the way to becoming a child, a state in which the influence of the conditioning factors of the environment, which we call **"echogenic"** factors, have a direct impact on the person (Fig. 1).

Modeling of our senses

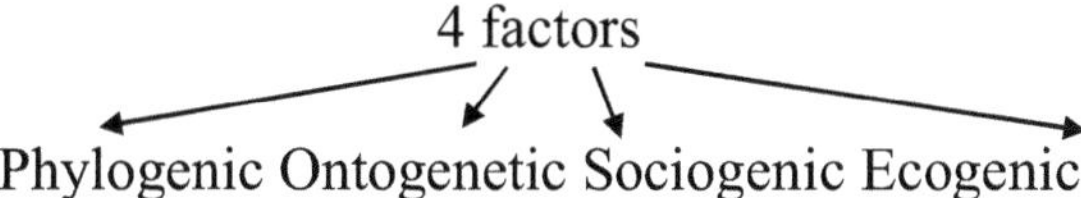

Fig. 1 Diagram of the factors that shape our senses

Each and every sense, including the sense of taste is shaped by these factors.

The senses, then, are in charge of capturing stimuli, but not all, but only those stimuli for which they are prepared to capture, in other words, the senses are the *first sensory filter* of human experiences. The only stimuli to which the human being has access are those for which he is sensitized, and there are only two types of stimuli: "Waves" and "Chemical substances".

Waves can be electromagnetic (light, color.), processed by the sense of sight, they can be pressure waves (sound, touch) processed by the senses of hearing and touch, we also have thermal waves (heat, cold) processed by the thermal receptors. In the group of chemical substances (smells, tastes) we have the processing by the senses of smell and taste. Outside these ways of perception, any other type of stimulus ceases to exist if there are no receptors and sensors to detect it.

The second sensory *filter* is in the **range of operability** that each sense has assigned to its function. Sight sees light and colors, some colors but not all, it cannot see infrared or ultraviolet, nor can it see all intensities.

Hearing captures sounds, but not all sounds, it cannot hear ultrasounds or infrasounds. Smell captures odors, but not all, and so on for each sense.

The third sensory *filter* is that the senses can only perceive **variations of stimuli**, for which they obviously have to be prepared. A constant stimulus is coded as null, non-existent. If a sound remains constant in intensity and frequency, it is no longer perceived as such (the brain ignores it), if a light has the same intensity and frequency, it is ignored, the same for touch, taste, etc.

If the sense has been activated, we can speak of emotions, understood as the broad set of stimuli and responses, which would be the *fourth* sensory *filter*. It is at this moment when we pass from the extra cranial to the intracranial phase, we pass from processes that occur outside the brain to processes that occur inside the brain. The first part, the extra cranial, is called **Transduction** and the second, which is intracranial, is called **Codification**.

In this phase the information (stimuli) captured by our senses travels through the various parts of the sensory organs without changing its meaning, so, for example, if we see the color blue, it remains blue as it goes through the various parts of the eyes. Transduction, therefore, takes place thanks to the presence of stimulus receptor structures[1,2] that connect with sensors that initiate the processing that will activate the senses. Once the organ of the stimulated sense has already been activated, the second phase called "Coding" begins, which is already intracranial and is characterized by the change of the interpretation of the information without modifying the means of transport, in this case the blue color changes in its meaning as it travels through the different parts of the brain becoming memories, sensations, ideas, projects, etc.[3,4] . Our brain is made up of one hundred billion neurons (currently it is considered that there are between 80 billion and 90 billion), whose main mission is to **reject 99% of the stimuli** we receive, since its optimal work is to use only 1% of all stimuli received, i.e. only 1% of what is received is taken into account. This brain requirement is the *fifth sensory filter*.

With this 1% the **predominant perception channels (**also called Modalities) **of** the person are activated; these channels are the senses. Each person has a system of unconscious sensory preferences, this makes that a certain person captures more easily information of visual type (is more prone to attend), or that another one captures better the auditory stimuli, others the internal sensations (Kinesthetic), and so on with the rest of senses. These channels are the *sixth sensory filter*. An example of this level can be seen in a hypothetical situation. Suppose that three people go to "contemplate" the "Concha de San Sebastian" , and each of them is asked how he/she would define the experience; it could happen that of the three people, one would say: "it is like a brushstroke of colors", another would explain that "it is like a waltz of the waves" and the third would answer: "it gives me the sensation of softness and warmth". Each of them would have seen the same scenario, but each of them would have let herself be subjugated by the most sensitive channel of her person; the first would have the visual channel, the second the auditory channel and the third the kinesthetic channel (inner sensation). We must specify that in real life there is no such purity of perception, there is a mixture with the predominance of one of them.

The *next filter, the seventh*, would be **feelings**. This filter makes the emotions**,** captured by the personal preferential channels, pass into feelings**.** Again, not all emotions give rise to feelings, but those that do will be the ones that will color our reasoning.

With emotions, feelings and reasoning we fully enter the territory of **communication**, which is the *eighth sensory filter*. We are used to understand that language is the main means of communication to connect concepts with words, allowing us to share thoughts, feelings (conceptualizations of emotions), knowledge, etc., but that is partially correct, since the usual verbal language communication only provides 7% of the total information, the remaining 93% is a-verbal, without words. In that a-verbality we find the tone of voice with 38% of participation, vision (eye movements, facial expressions, body movements, postures, etc.) with 55%. Other senses complement communication: taste, smell and touch. In other words, all these forms of communication end up transformed into emotions, feelings and reasons in the receiver.

Communication (we exchange information), implies that "ideas" arise, which will give rise to "beliefs", which will build our "criteria", which will shape our "values" which become the beacons that each person puts to mark his path, stimulating him to pay attention to the characteristics of the path he has taken. These values form "attitudes" that will create **"habits",** which will be *the ninth level of a* person's sensory *filter*,

The *tenth level of* sensory *filter*, appears when the information that has reached the brain is stored **(memory)** in two different areas, the **conscious** area that only collects 10% of the data and the **unconscious** area that collects 90% of the data, even in coma states[5] .

The *eleventh filter level* is the personal **medical history** (health status). Nothing that does not happen is left out of our clinical history.

We have more filters, but we will only expose one last filter, *the twelfth filter* called **Chronobiosensory**, constituted by the variations in the sensitivity of a living organism to capture stimuli, depending on time (time of day, month, season, age, etc.[6] . This filter makes all the previous levels depend on these moments, on these temporalities. This pattern-base is important to understand the fact that our sensations and perceptions are part of a scarce amount of information to which we are allowed to have access, as a consequence of the different filters that have been acting constantly, reducing the information according to the properties that each filter is able to manage. The filters not only reshape the events that reach us but also discard what they cannot manage (Fig. 2).

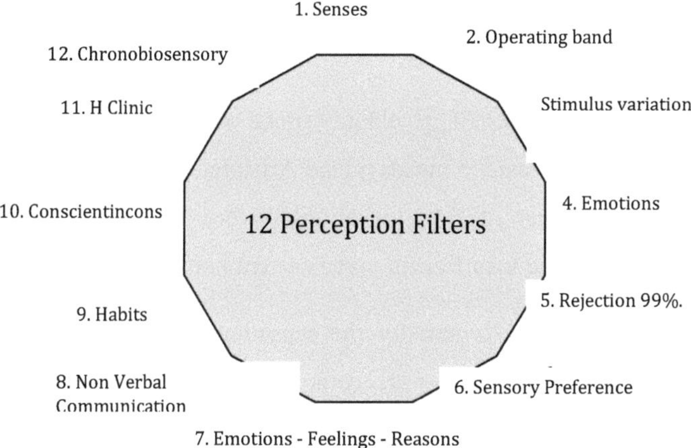

Fig.2. The 12 filters that build our perception

If we ask ourselves what is the link between the filters and the sense of taste, the answer should be: to understand that the set of filters is the framework where the construction of the sensory perception of taste takes place. To get an idea, you only have to think of a taste experience, whatever it may be, and apply each of the filters, and discover how it is influenced according to the characteristics of each filter.

2-The sense of taste (structures)-

All of the above is modeling the perception of taste. However, we have not defined what we should understand as "perception". Perception must be understood as the moment when we become "conscious" of our sensations. Thus, we only have perception of taste when we become aware of the sensation of taste.

The sense of taste, being part of the twelve filters of perception, has an extra-cranial phase that we call Transduction, followed by an intracranial phase called Coding.

Aristotle (384-322 BC.)[7] already spoke of pungent taste, aggressive taste and astringent taste. Nowadays, the Aristotelian tendency to consider taste as the manager of four sensations (sweet, bitter, sour and salty) continues, both being insufficient, given current knowledge.

What is certain is that for the sensation and perception of taste, human beings have structures (receptors) that are mainly located in the tongue, palate, pharynx, epiglottis and larynx[8] , which are called taste buds, of which we have about 5000 (Fig.3) and which are responsible for discriminating tastes.

5000 taste buds

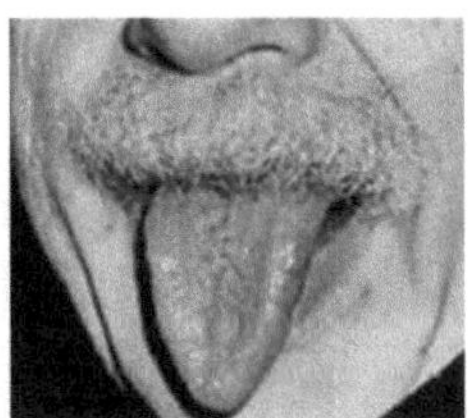

Language

Soft palate

Pharynx

Epiglottis

Larynx

Fig., 3 Distribution of taste buds.

Within these buttons are 50 to 100 types of specialized cells with sensors that detect sweet, salty, sour, bitter and other tastes such as umami, kokumi, etc. (Fig. 4 and 5).

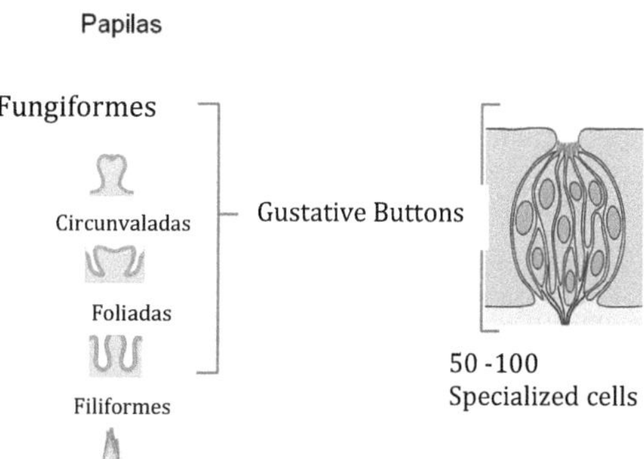

Fig.4. Different types of papillae with taste buds.
Of the four types of papillae, only the filiform papillae are not usually have taste buds.

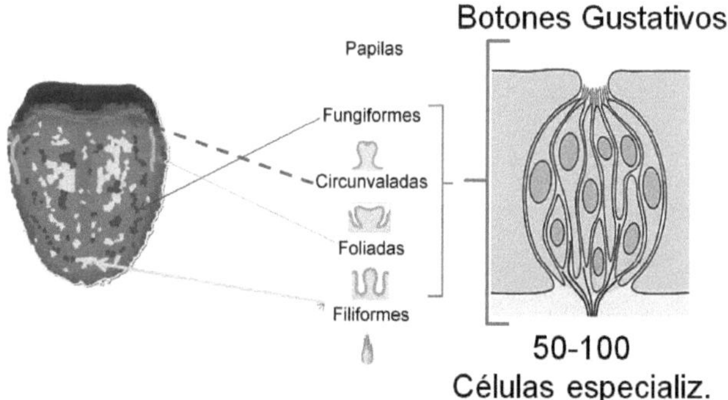

Fig. 5. Location of the papillae. The taste buds are more or less evenly distributed throughout the tongue, with areas of greater density.

Taste implies the presence of taste buds that are connected to nerves called Cranial nerves V (Trigeminal), VII (Facial), IX (Glossopharyngeal), X (Vagus) and XII[9] (Hypoglossal) that do not participate in the taste, but in the movement of the tongue (Fig.6). (Fig. 6).) that have to conduct the stimulus to the brain, these nerves have other functions, therefore, the gustatory sensation is not a perception restricted to the 4 classic tastes (sweet, salty, sour, etc.) but we must add the other actions that these nerves perform, in addition to the perceptions of all the other senses, also called modalities or channels, such as: touch (analyzes the degree of softness, the degree of dryness, viscosity, hardness, temperature, itching, etc.), pain (the degree of discomfort, the degree of pain, the degree of pain, the degree of pain, the degree of pain, the degree of pain, the degree of pain, the degree of pain, the degree of pain, the degree of pain, the degree of pain, the degree of pain, the degree of pain, the degree of pain, the degree of pain, the degree of pain, etc.).), pain (degree of discomfort), motor perception (mobility, ability and coordination) of the linguo-maxillo-oropharyngeal movements essential for palatability and swallowing[10] , of what is tasted, to finally take into account the neurovegetative perception (which regulates the thresholds of sensitivity of the five tastes), and finally the neurovegetative perception (which regulates the thresholds of sensitivity of the five tastes, Finally, the neurovegetative perception (which regulates the sensitivity thresholds of the five tastes, as well as touch, pain, and movement, which are captured by the different nerve fibers of the cranial nerves that connect with the taste buds) must be taken into account.

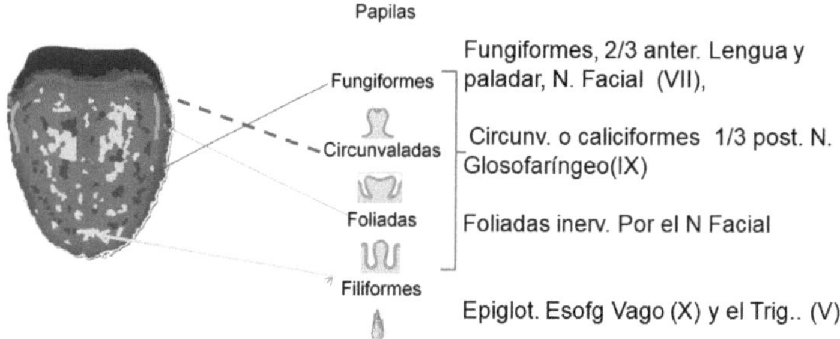

Fig. 6. Location of the papillae and their innervation.

We have 50 genes dedicated to taste and smell[11] , which confer sapid perceptions that are much broader than the classic five tastes. Each of these tastes is encoded differently, thus sweet taste is encoded via G-protein, while salty perception is managed by sodium ion exchange (Na $)^{+}$ which, interestingly enough, acts on the channels for Amiloride, which is an antihypertensive. Acid perception is handled by Na^{+} o/ and potassium ion exchange (K^{+}), bitter perception is handled by a combination of K^{+} ion exchange and G-protein (mostly)[12] , while for umami[13] it is carried out via Glutamate receptors. That said, as generic as it may seem, we must keep in mind that people can present different taste patterns, which have been genetically encoded[14] . The place where these phenomena occur is in the cells inside the taste buds (Fig. 5).

Within these buttons there are three main types of receptor cells that activate certain perceptions. We have Type I cells that manage the salty taste, Type II cells for umami, sweet and bitter taste, and Type III cells for acid taste.(Fig.7).

Células especializadas
Tipo I (Salado)
Tipo II (Umami, Dulce, Amargo)
Tipo III (Ácido)

Fig.7 Different cell types for different tastes.

Type I and Type III receptor cells are involved in the detection of salty and sour tastes, which act via ion channels, while Type III cells detect sweet, bitter and umami tastes, whose action is carried out via membrane proteins called "**G-protein-coupled receptors,** via their nerves VII, IX, while spicy, pungent, hot, burning and cold are handled by the trigeminal nerve (V) and the movement of the tongue by the hypoglossal nerve (XII).

3-The sense of taste (receptors)-.

The receptor cells that we have described in the previous chapter, present a whole series of sensory receptors that are involved in the detection of the different tastes, this type of sensory receptors are called TAS1R1, TAS1R3 TAS1R2, TAS1R3, TAS2Rs, PKD2L1, PKD1L3, TRPs and TRPV1, TRPM8, TRPA1. The distribution of all of them, throughout the oropharynx, leads to certain sensory predominances.

There are not only these, there are more tastes that are appearing that produce generation of taste perception, in fact there are many more receptors but they are not included in this list because they are not linked to the taste system.

Let us look at each of the receptors as they are linked to the different taste perceptions such as savory taste, also called umami, which is like a sweet-sour perception, sweet taste, bitter taste, salty taste, spicy taste, cold taste, pungent spicy taste, burning spicy taste, cold taste, and fatty taste. In Fig. 8 we can see the different types of sensations, as well as why they have been given these names.

Tipos de Receptores del Gusto

- **Umami** ;TAS1R1 (Taste Receptor Type 1, member 1)
  TAS1R3 (Taste Receptor Type 1, member 3)

- **Dulce**:TAS1R2 (taste receptor type 1, member 2)
  TAS1R3 (taste receptor type 1, member 3)

- **Amargo**:25 tipos de TAS2Rs (taste receptor type 2)

- **Salado:** PKD2L1 (polycystic kidney disease 1)
  PKD1L3, (polycystic kidney disease 3)

- **Picante quemante** (Capsaicina): TRPs y TRPV1

- **Frío**: (Mentol, Alcanfor,Etanol) TRPM8

- **Picante pungente**:(Aceite Mostaza, Wasabi, Rábano picante, ajo) TRPA1

- **Grasa.** Posible Receptor CD36, GPR120 Y GPR40

Fig. 8. We can observe the different receptors and the Anglo-Saxon origin of their names that each receptor has. Each of the 3 cell types (I, II, and III) have, depending on their function, different taste receptors.

These different receptors are found in the cell membrane of the three types of cells for taste.[15] (Fig.9).

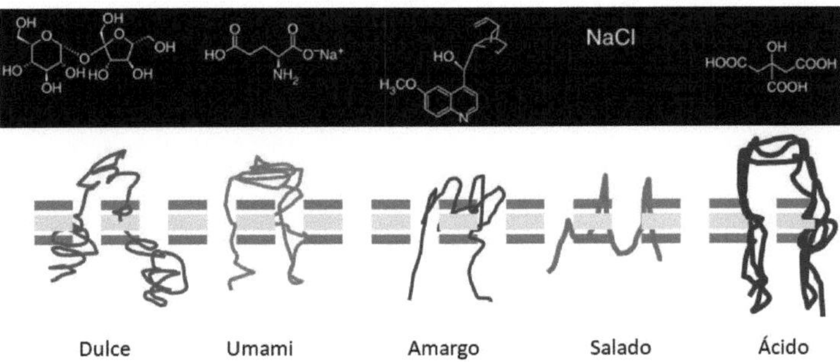

Fig. 9, Representation of how the receptors cross the cell membrane, which is why they are called "Transmembrane Receptors". The inner part of the cell is where each receptor begins and ends, while the outer part is where the receptor is contacted by the external stimulus.

New tastes have been discovered. Fig.10 and 11a show the 13 tastes that are currently taken into account and the substances that produce them.

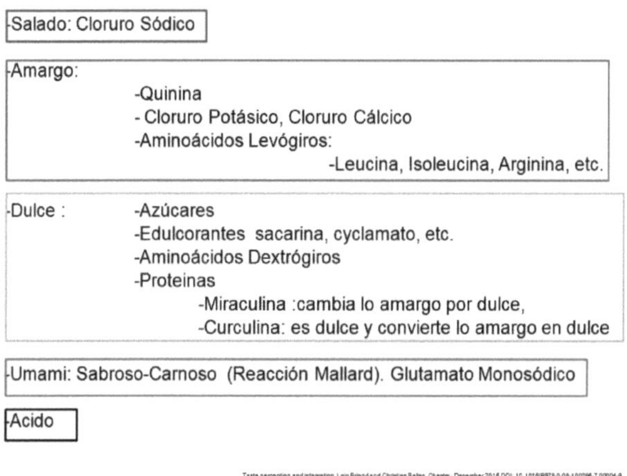

Fig.10

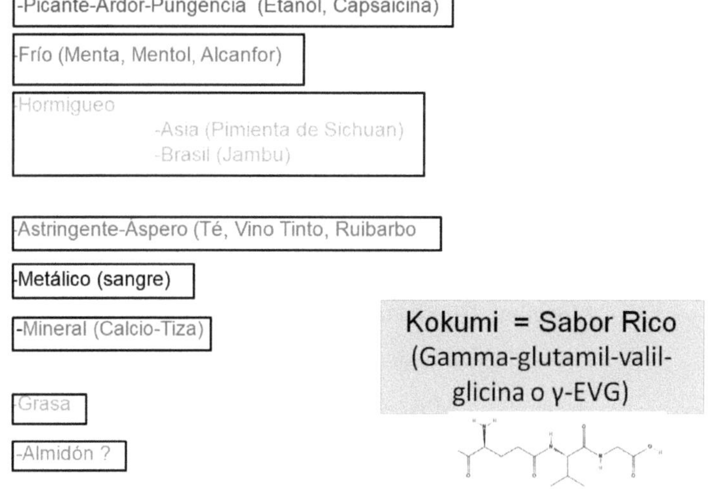

Fig.11a

Not all the exposed tastes have their sensory receptors confirmed. There are tastes that are described verbally, based on sensations, without having yet been discovered whether or not they have their corresponding sensory receptors. And to complicate things further, we must know that there are different substances that produce the same taste effect, for example:

-Salt we have Sodium Chloride, Calcium, Potassium, Lithium, Ammonium,

-For **Bitter**:

-Quinine

- Potassium Chloride, Calcium Chloride

-Levorotatory Amino Acids:

Leucine, Isoleucine, Valine, Arginine,
Methionine, Phenylalanine, Tyrosine, Tryptophan, Histidine

-For **the sweet taste**:

-Sugars

-Sweeteners (saccharin, cyclamate, acesulfamate-K, aspartame, neotame, advantame, sucralose, etc.)

-Dextrorotatory amino acids -Proteins such as Taumatin, Monellin, Brazzein, Pentadin, Miraculin (changes bitter to sweet), Neoculin or Curculin is sweet and turns bitter to sweet)

-Umami: MSG, IMP, GMP, Mallard reaction

-Kokumi (fullness of mouth)

-Acid: Acids

There are other tastes, which are under study, apart from the classics, such as:

-Spicy-burning-burning-heat. Substances such as ethanol and capsaicin from hot bell pepper, piperine from black pepper, gingerol from ginger root and allyl isothiocyanate from horseradish.
-The **spicy-cold-fresh**. Such as peppermint, spearmint menthol, anethole, ethanol and camphor.

But also other perceptions such as:

-Numbness, tingling (Sichuan pepper, chili bell pepper and jambu).

-Astringent-harsh as tea, red wine or rhubarb.

Metallic[16,17] produced by chemical reactions between substances, by drugs or by taste alterations.

-Calcium taste, Calcium receptors are known in the animal world.

-Taste Fat. Possible taste receptor called CD36[18] located on circumvallate and foliate taste buds).[22]and possible G protein-coupled receptors GPR120 and GPR40.

-Starch taste. It has been suggested that humans can taste starch (specifically, a glucose oligomer) independently of other tastes such as sweet. **However, no specific chemical receptor for this** taste **has yet been found**.

-Full flavor. Kokumi, which means "full flavor" or "rich" and describes food compounds that have no flavor of their own, but enhance characteristics when combined, even enhances umami. Thus, alongside the five basic tastes of sweet, sour, salty, salty, bitter, *kokumi'* has been described as something that can enhance the other five tastes by broadening and prolonging the other tastes, and thus the "mouthfeel".

This set of perceptions shows us that the concept of taste is an extraordinarily broad territory. We can already see that it is not so much the lack of a vocabulary as the lack of its use that is at fault.

Having explained the basic elements, we must point out that the classical territories of taste, where the language is divided into areas of taste localization, are now an anachronistic concept (Fig. 11b). To understand this anachronism we have to enter into the expanded and even extended vision of the sense of taste.

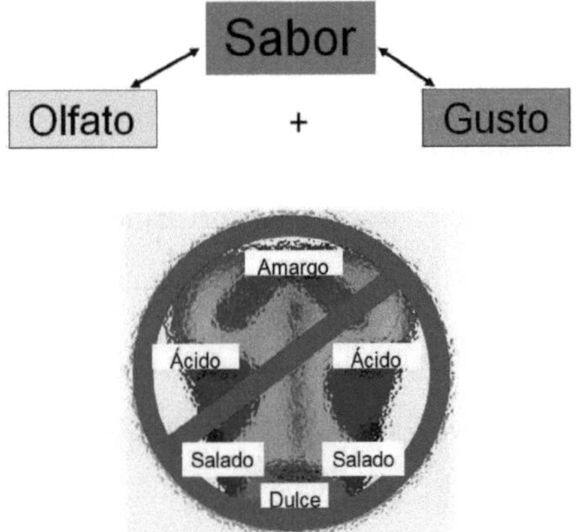

Fig. 11b. Classical areas of taste localization, which are no longer meaningful.

4-Extended view of Taste-

Taste, which is responsible for the management of sweetness, saltiness, sourness, bitterness, umami, and others, as we have already explained, is supported, in the first instance, by sapidity (palatability) constituted by the presence of "other" senses, apart from taste. These other senses are touch (texture, temperature, hydration, etc.), pain, sound, color, the receptors of the neurovegetative system (sympathetic and parasympathetic) and the motor nervous system, to which must be added the taste perceptions that are known today. Moreover, this "sapid" system that we have described, together with the sense of smell, is part of what we call taste. Taste is the conjugation of the Sapid and the Aroma (the smell of what is eaten and ingested). The sapid must be understood as the set of perceptions that appear in the mouth that are not part of the world of smell. The aroma is the odorous structuring that is influenced by the sapid action of what penetrates our mouth, and that via retronasal, when swallowing, penetrates the nose and activates the olfactory system where we also find the same "other" perceptions produced by the same "other" senses that participate in the construction of taste, but that are now in the nostrils, unlike those of taste that are in the mouth (fig. 12,13a, and 13b).

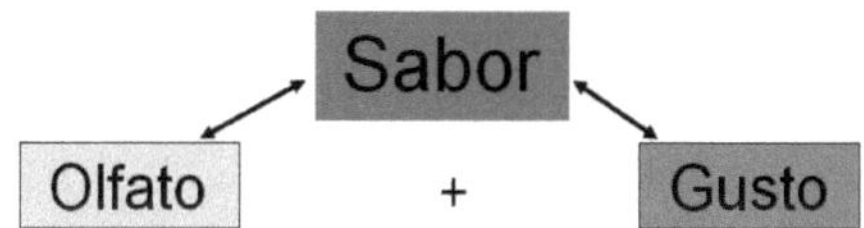

Fig.12. Taste is constructed by Smell and Taste.

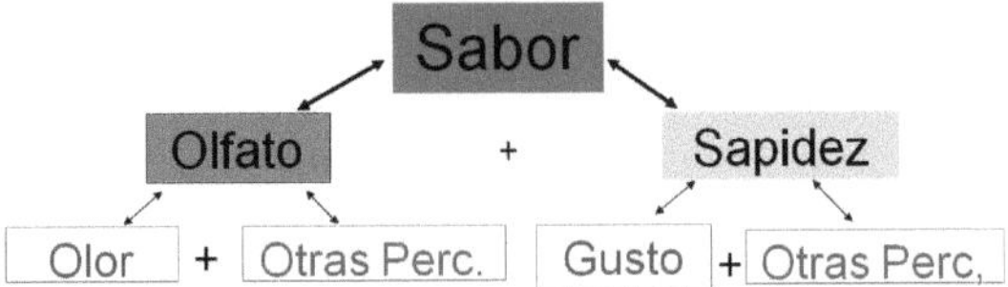

Fig. 13(a) As we can see, olfaction captures smell and other perceptions, while sapidity captures taste and other perceptions as well.

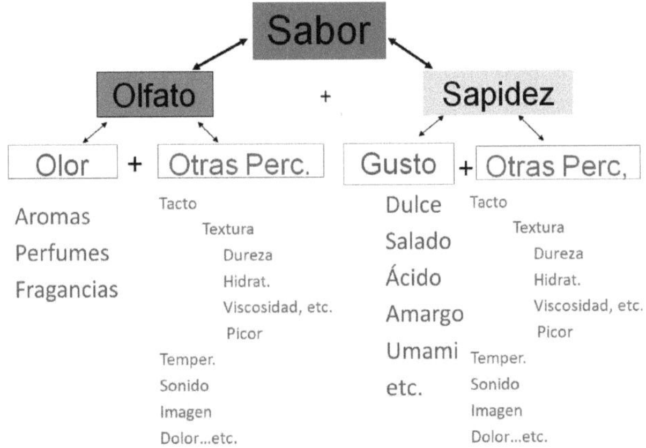

Fig.13(b) Enlarged view of the characteristics of each of the parts of the taste, where the taste is located.

This type of format in which one sense is influenced by the other senses, we call it "Polymodal", in fact, all senses are Polymodal, that is to say, each one of the senses depends on the other senses, here we will focus on the analysis of taste from the Polymodal vision. The nerves involved in this polymodality, as we have already indicated, are called Cranial nerves. We will start with the receptors of touch, spiciness and pain[19] , which we will discuss in the next chapter....

5-The sense of touch and spicy -

We are used to understand that taste is sweet, salty, sour and bitter, but there are other perceptions such as pain and spiciness (Fig.14)....

Receptores Tacto y Dolor

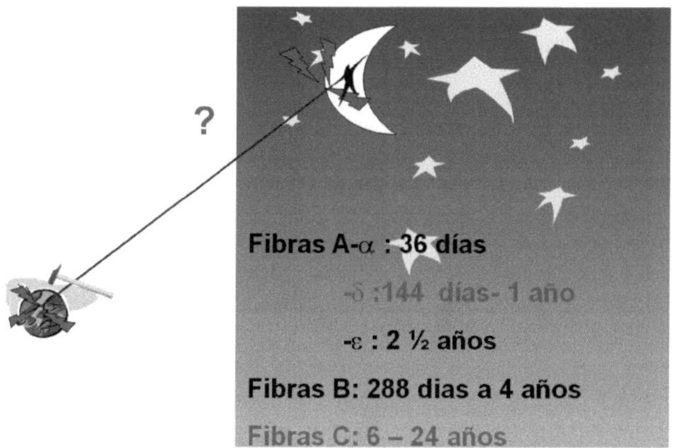

Fig.14. Nerve fibers transmitting pain and their comparative velocity.

The receptors and fibers that transmit pain are the A-Delta (δ) fibers, which are myelinic and transmit the impulse 4-30 mts/sec, and the C myelinic fibers, which are more abundant and transmit more slowly, 0.4-2mts/sec. and the C-myelinic fibers, which are the most abundant, transmit more slowly, 0.4-2mts/sec. We can see in Fig. 14 the differences in transmission speed assuming the case of a person who was on the Moon and one of the arms was so long that his hand was on the Earth. If someone with a hammer hit that hand, the person would perceive the pain and its characteristics at different times, for example, for the A-δ fibers it would take 144 days to 1 year to perceive the type of pain they generate, while the type C fibers would take between 6 and 24 years to give the sensation in the type of pain they produce.

Researchers who have recently contributed information on pain and touch receptors are the 2021 Nobel Laureates in Medicine Ardem Patapoutian and David Julius (Fig. 15). Ardem and Julius contributed new research, along separate lines, on pain from thermal, mechanical, chemical, burning, and touch causes.

Premios Nobel 2021

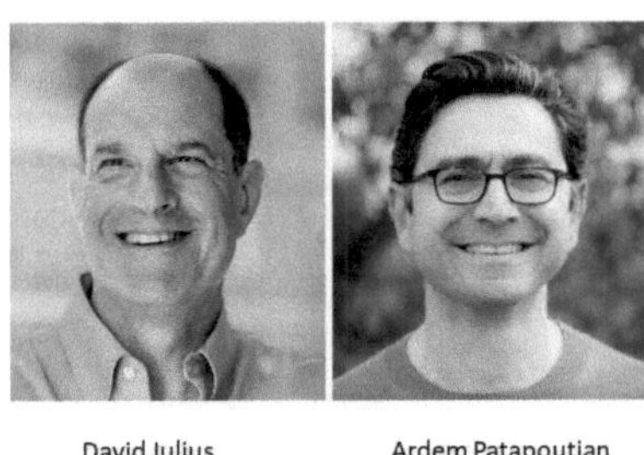

David Julius Ardem Patapoutian

Fig. 15. https://www.bbc.com/mundo/noticias-58787574

Ardem Patapoutian is a Lebanese-born Armenian molecular biologist who emigrated to the U.S. In 2021 (age 56) he received the Nobel Prize in Medicine and Physiology jointly with David Julius for his discoveries in temperature and touch receptors. He works at the Scripps Research Institute. Patapoutian did an experiment that led to the discovery of a different type of receptor that is activated in response to mechanical force or touch.

David Julius is an American biochemist and is 66 years old. Currently a professor at the University of California in San Francisco, he found that there is a receptor (a part of our cells that detects what is around it) that responded to capsaicin, which is also found in hot peppers. Further tests showed that the receptor responded to heat and was activated when there were temperatures that caused "pain".

In turn Julius and Patapoutian found a receptor that could detect cold. Another finding was that they found that the heat sensor TRPV1 was involved in chronic pain and how our body regulated core temperature. They also found that the tactile receptor PIEZ02 had multiple functions, such as participating in micturition (urination function) or participating in blood pressure regulation. It has also been found, for example, that the TRPA1 receptor participates in sneezing and cough reflexes.[20,] This shows clearly how the same receptor participates in different functions (Fig. 16). This aspect has a relevant importance, since it implies a new vision of the concept of sense and sensory-receptor. The fact that a sense has more functions than expected and that it is found in more places than expected suggests the existence of actions that break the rigid scheme that the senses have always had, which is why all sensoriality must be rethought, as we will explain later on.

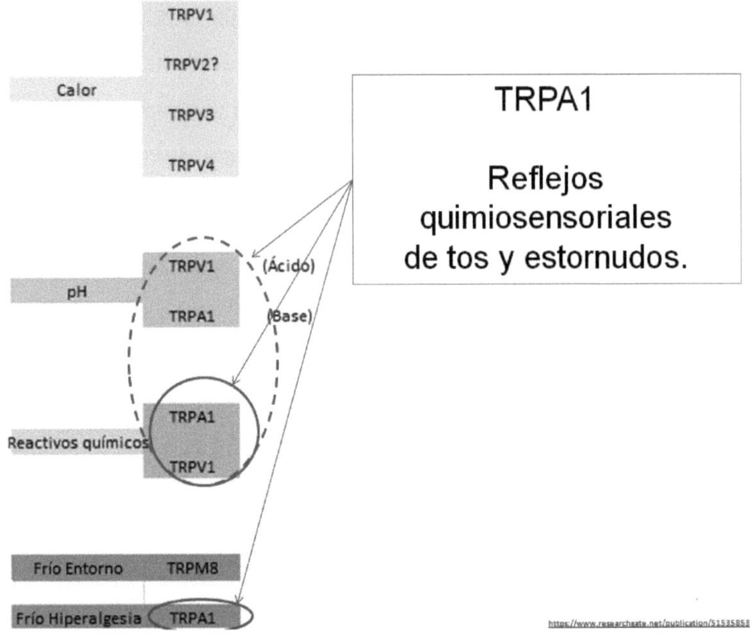

Fig.16. Different TRP receptors[21] at different sensory sites.

One of the receptors responsible for the perception of heat and spiciness is capsaicin (Fig. 17).

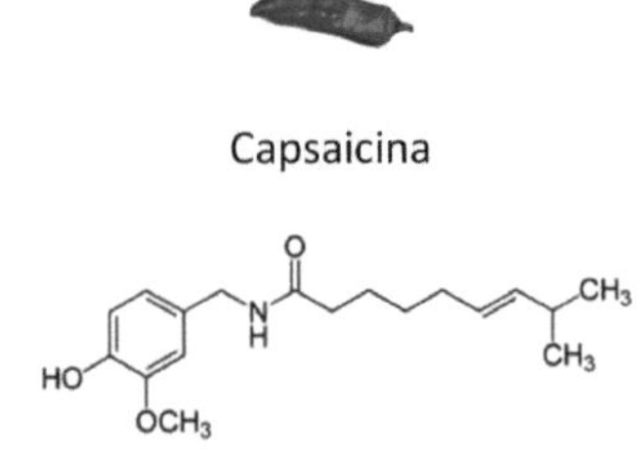

Fig.17. Capsaicin is found in chili and jalapeño peppers.

David Julius' discovery of TRPV1 receptors for temperature provided insight into how temperature differences can induce electrical signals in the nervous system.[22] This type of receptor is again shown to be involved in various functions, as we have already seen in Fig. 16 and can see in Fig. 18.

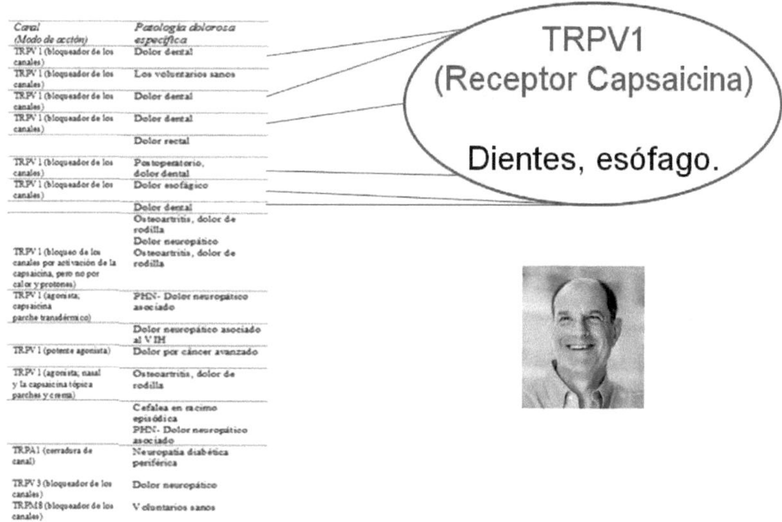

Canal (Modo de acción)	*Patología dolorosa específica*
TRPV1 (bloqueador de los canales)	Dolor dental
TRPV1 (bloqueador de los canales)	Los voluntarios sanos
TRPV1 (bloqueador de los canales)	Dolor dental
TRPV1 (bloqueador de los canales)	Dolor dental
	Dolor rectal
TRPV1 (bloqueador de los canales)	Postoperatorio, dolor dental
TRPV1 (bloqueador de los canales)	Dolor esofágico
	Dolor dental
TRPV1 (bloqueo de los canales por activación de la capsaicina, pero no por calor y protones)	Osteoartritis, dolor de rodilla Dolor neuropático Osteoartritis, dolor de rodilla
TRPV1 (agonista; capsaicina parche tranadérmico)	PHN- Dolor neuropátsco asociado
	Dolor neuropático asociado al VIH
TRPV1 (potente agonista)	Dolor por cáncer avanzado
TRPV1 (agonista; nasal y la capsaicina tópica parches y crema)	Osteoartritis, dolor de rodilla
	Cefalea en racimo episódica PHN- Dolor neuropático asociado
TRPA1 (cerradura de canal)	Neuropatía diabética periférica
TRPV3 (bloqueador de los canales)	Dolor neuropático
TRPM8 (bloqueador de los canales)	Voluntarios sanos

Fig.18. We can observe that a receptor, which in principle had the function of detecting thermal and painful stimuli of the skin, we see them in other parts of the body affecting other totally different functions (*Ana Gabriela Medina Torres (Algology, INCMNSZ). Bibliographic Review: Nociceptive TRP channels in multiple pain pathologies).*

Recall that we are talking about transmembrane receptors (Fig. 9 and 19). A transmembrane receptor, as described in Fig. 9, is a chemical structure that crosses the cell membrane from the inside to the outside and then penetrates back into the cell from the outside to the inside. The extracellular zone of this structure is the part where the (taste) stimulus activates the receptor, triggering the taste sensation.

TRPV1

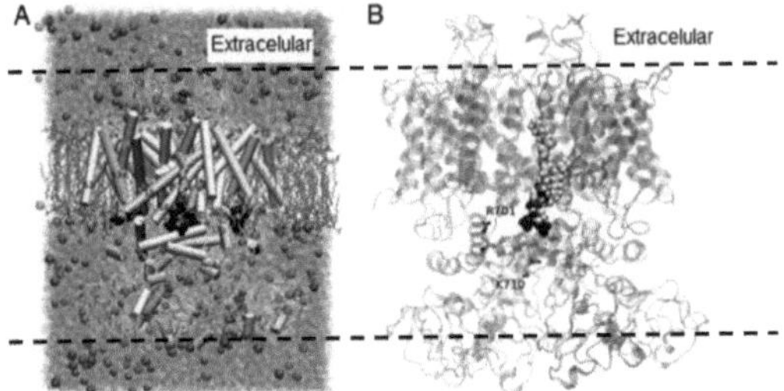

Arrangement of the TRPV1-type transmembrane receptor structures[23] .

Julius and Patapoutian used the chemical menthol (Fig. 20) to identify the sensory receptor TRPM8, which was activated by cold. Other ion channels were also identified, but this time related to TRPV1 and TRPM8, and were found to be activated at different temperatures.

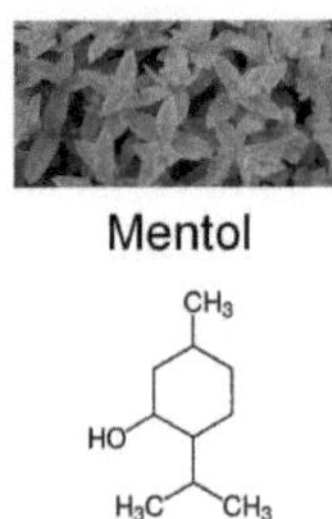

Fig. 20. Chemical structure of menthol.

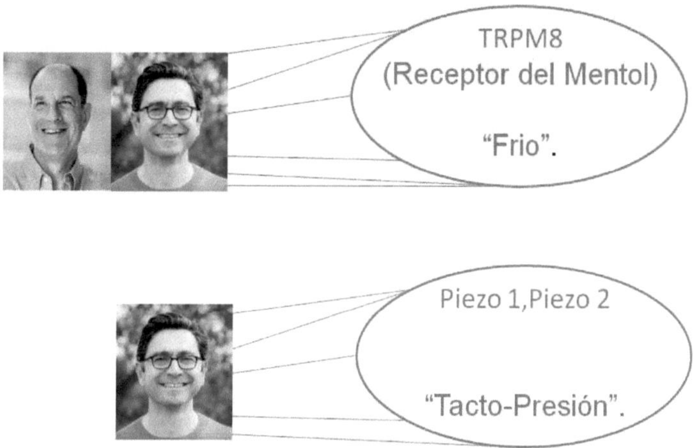

Fig.21. Receptors investigated by the two nobel prizes.

Patapoutian discovered two mechano-sensitive ion channels that he named Piezo1 (Piezo means pressure in Greek) and Piezo2 (Fig. 21), which are activated by pressure on the cell and are involved in the sensation of touch, position detection and movement.

There is a great variety of TRP-type channels such as TRPV1-4, TRPA1, TRPM2, TRPM4-5, TRPM8 and TRPC5 that encode thermal (for temperature, for the hot sensation of spicy and the cold sensation of menthol), chemical (pain) and mechanical stimuli. They have also been shown to participate in other functions such as thermoregulation, salivary secretion, inflammation, cardiovascular regulation, smooth muscle tone, calcium and magnesium homeostasis. Piezo sensors (Piezo1 and 2) have been found to be involved in touch (Piezo1), blood pressure, respiration, bladder control of urine and body position and movement[24] (Fig.22).

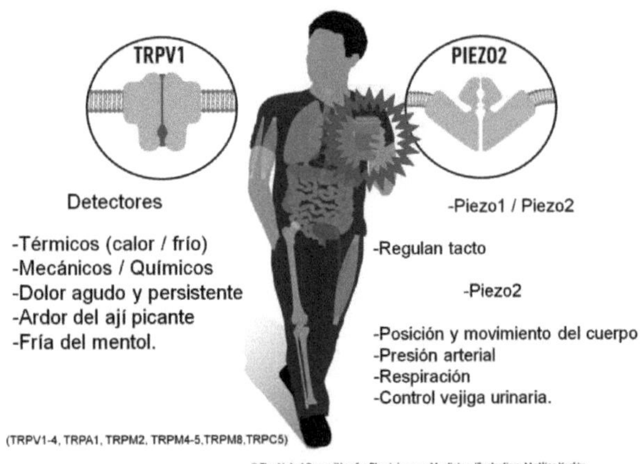

Fig. 22. Actions of the different receptors[25] .

6-The "Panubication" of the taste receptors.

It has been shown that taste receptors are not only found in the territories of the mouth and pharynx, but can also be found in adipose tissue (fats), macrophages, airways and nasosinusal cavities, trachea and bronchi, gastrointestinal tract, pancreas[26] , testes[27] , an example of which are the bitter taste sensory receptors in the skin[28] .

It has been shown that the bitter taste receptors T2R38 also regulate the mucosal defenses of the upper respiratory tract. This type of receptor detects bacterial toxic secretions, which not only act in the lungs but also in the sinus cavities in the presence of sinusitis, and it has even been discovered that these receptors are activated in situations of hyperglycemia[29,30] .

Olfactory receptors have also been found, in this case, in the brain, skin, eyes, musculature, airways, lungs, heart, liver, spleen, kidneys, pancreas, colon, enterochromaffin cells, bladder, prostate, testicles, blood, skeletal muscle. [31, 32]

How important are these receptors in the world of taste?

It is surprising to discover that what we always took for granted about the sensory receptors of our body, that is to say that we only found them exercising a concrete and specific function in each organ such as the cones and rods in the eyes, taste buds on the tongue, temperature, pressure, in the skin, olfactory cells in the nose, etc., today we know that it is no longer so, since such sensory receptors can be found in various places of our body, participating in functions totally different from those that were exclusively supposed to them.

However, what is most disturbing is not the above, but the intuition that if these sensory sensors are capable of participating in different functions, the question arises: are they not already carrying out these functions, which are different from those we have usually understood, in the places where they have always been exclusively located?

In other words, it could happen, for example, that an olfactory sensor (located in the nose) or a taste sensor (located in the mouth) could also be managing pulmonary, renal, cardiac functions, etc. already from their classical location that corresponds to them by the fact of being activated by odors or tastes. But there is more, we could suspect that these receptors, distributed by the different organs of our body, could be activated by classical stimuli belonging to them, for example taste receptors located in the intestine can be activated by contacting them with certain tastes; or that odor receptors located in the lungs are activated by developing a function other than the classical olfactory one.

These conjectures have ceased to be so, since at present, what we have described as possible actions are happening as such.

We are seeing what it means to discover taste receptors. We have made reference to the respiratory system, among others, and as we are in the territory of taste, we enter the digestive system, appropriate territory of the world of taste and its influences. We take as an example the enteroendocrine system (cellular set) distributed throughout the digestive system, which connects with the sensory system[33] , and therefore are part of the taste, insofar as their linkage modifies the "appetite" of a nutrient, a food or a meal for the person. This allows us, for example, to understand the existence of the preference of sugar over sweeteners[34] , and also helps us to understand that certain odors can be understood as aromas, since let us remember that flavor is, in short, [(taste + smell) x touch]. Or the effects of sandalwood (Fig. 23) on capillary tissue regeneration[35] , or its effect on leukemia by reducing it[36] .

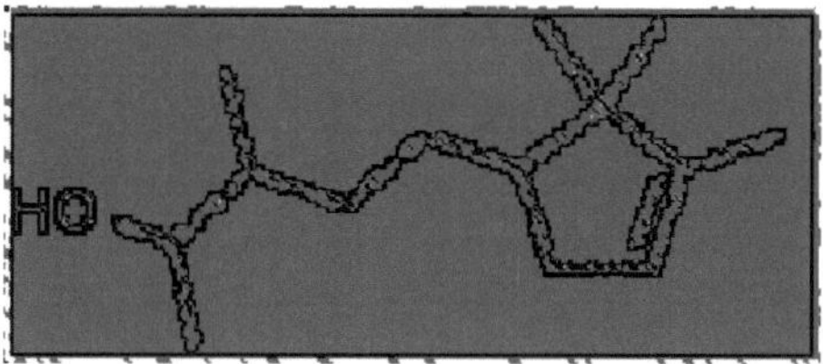

Fig. 23. Sandalore structure

Or, for example, the dysphagic effects (alteration of swallowing) produced by covid[37] and the action of certain aromas and odors such as menthol, which favors swallowing by increasing the frequency of swallowing by reducing the time between swallowing and swallowing, an effect that cold water (23º) has, but to a lesser degree than menthol[38] .

Such a similar effect is found with cinnamon through cinnamaldehyde (organic compound responsible for the taste and characteristic odor of cinnamon); which associated with $ZnSO_4$ (zinc sulfate) increases the frequency of swallowing[39] (Fig.24).

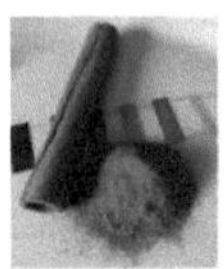

Cinamaldehido

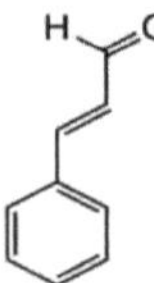

Fig. 24. Cinnamon as an adjuvant for swallowing

Touch is another component of taste. One of the ways to activate tastes is by means of electric lingual touch. Thus, for example, there is the possibility of enhancing taste, without increasing the presence of chemical substances, or even reducing their presence, such as the perception of salty taste with very low concentrations of sodium chloride in food, or of other tastes, all achieved by means of electronic stimulators, as in the case of the designs made by Professor Dr. Homei Miyashita of Meijii University in Japan, which achieve, by means of electronic stimulators, the perception of salty taste with very low concentrations of sodium chloride in food, or of other tastes. Homei Miyashita of the Meijii University of Japan, who uses common food utensils (glasses, bowls, plates, chopsticks), to which he has connected very low intensity current systems to increase these perceptions.[40, 41] This is a technology that could be described as reality-enhancing (Fig. 25 and 26).

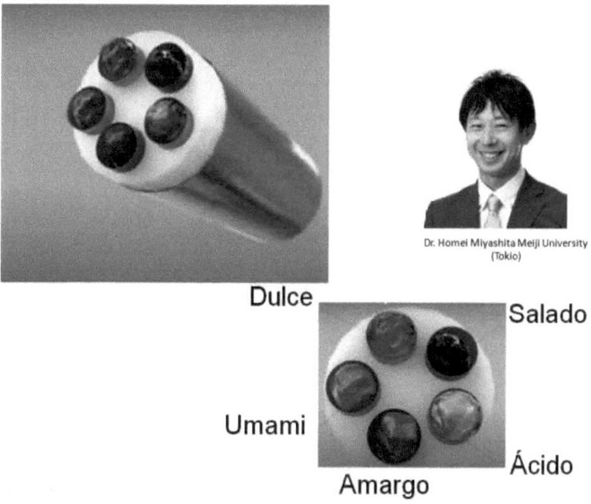

Fig. 25. Design of Dr. Homei Miyashita's taste stimulator, which when placed on the tongue can perceive the different tastes.

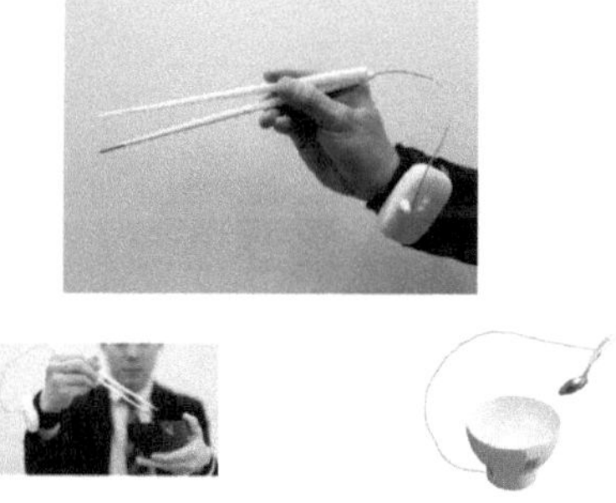

Dr. Homei Miyashita's design of electrostimulated chopsticks. These chopsticks are connected to a battery, whose circuit is connected to the bowl where the food is, and which is held in the other hand, closing the circuit when the food is placed in the mouth.

7-Transgusto, Gestated Taste, Microbiome and Pharmaceuticals.

We have some new aspects and concepts about the world of taste such as "Transtaste", "Gestated Taste" Microbiome and "Pharmaco-Taste" (Fig.27).

-Transgusto

-Gusto Gestado

-Microbioma

-Farmaco-Gusto

Fig. 27 New dimensions of taste and flavor

What do we mean by transtaste? Transtaste consists of keeping in mind the perception that the senses other than taste contribute to taste. If we were to make the experience of annulling all the senses except taste, we would realize the poverty of the sense of taste by isolating it from the other senses. We have explained that taste is part of flavor, which is constructed by combining the action of the other senses. If we imagine putting a piece of apple in our mouth, we can realize that it has a shape (vision), a smell (smell), it has a hardness, a weight, a temperature (touch) and it generates a noise, a sound (chewing, insalivation). In other words, taste, which is part of flavor, depends for its proper function, on the participation of the other senses. To the extent that the other senses, and not only the sense of taste, are altered, taste is modified. We can vary the taste by modifying the other aspects that participate in the other senses. If we stain a white wine to make it look like a red wine, it will be perceived as red wine, if, with our eyes covered, we remove (annul) the crunchy sound of potato chips, by applying a sound in our ears that does not allow us to hear the crunching of the chips, we will not identify that they are chips when we put them in our mouth and chew them. But this does not happen only with taste, but also with the other senses in relation to each other. This means that not only the sense of taste, but all the senses are co-constructed and depend on each other.

It becomes evident that the concept of transtaste consists of taste that navigates through the other senses, being impregnated with the characteristics of all the other senses, it is therefore a Codification, as we described it in the introduction of this book.

If we delve even deeper into the world of the senses, what else will we discover? We will discover that to the territory of the five classic senses, we have to add at least 5 more senses. These other senses are: Balance, Pain, Pressure, Concentration and the Chronobiological sense; so we can say that we have 10 senses (Fig.28).

¿Qué descubriremos más?

10-Sentidos

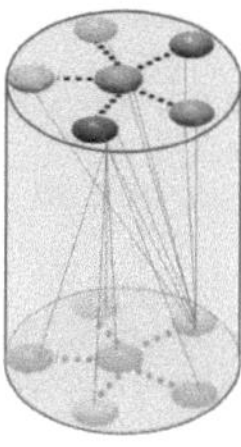

Fig. 28 We have more than 5 senses, we have 10 senses that are interconnected and influence each other.

If we try to describe these other five senses we will find that; The sense of balance is the one that allows us to know the stability of our body and its displacement (if it is immobile, if it turns to one side or another, if it accelerates, if it brakes, goes up, goes down, goes forward or backward, etc.).

The sense of pain informs us of structural and/or functional alterations of the body.

The sense of pressure is responsible for detecting the pressure exerted by matter in its three usual states (solid, liquid and gas), or what is the same, the pressure exerted by all solid matter ingested by us, such as the volume of food in our stomach, the same happens with the incorporation of liquids in our body, as happens in the urine bladder when it is full, or blood pressure, and in the case of the pressure exerted by gases in our body, at the pulmonary, gastric and intestinal level. These are just a few examples.

If we look at the direction of the concentrations, we must also consider

also enter the three states of matter, solid, liquid and gas, as would be the case of the concentration of salts in our body, of hormones such as insulin, of neurotransmitters such as dopamine, and in liquids we would have the dissolution of glucose, or of proteins, while in gases it would be the concentration of oxygen, carbon dioxide, nitrogen, etc.

Last but not least, we have the Chronobiological sense, which is in charge of regulating our biological clock. This sense tells us at what time of the day we are and therefore which functions are more important to carry out at each moment, since our body modifies its sensoriality according to the hours of the day, month, season and age.

In short, and in other words, each of these five other senses influences and modifies the capacities of the other five senses, among them: taste. In fact, there are more senses than we have exposed here, but we are not going to talk about them in order not to complicate the understanding of taste, but we can already say that the sense of taste is a "Multisensory Transtaste".

If we go one step further, and taking up the thread of one of the filters mentioned in the first chapter, we can see that the construction of the sense of taste takes place during gestation, based on this knowledge we can describe the influence of the mother on the future person in the embryonic and fetal stages of gestation with respect to taste. Therefore, taste is one of those territories that are influenced (educated) by maternal appetites and influences while we are being gestated. *Taste*, which begins its development before smell, is capable of distinguishing different nuances that we obtain in our intake of amniotic fluid. This function is performed by means of the taste buds found on our tongue, palate, throat, esophagus and even larynx. Thanks to these papillae we distinguish, for example, between sweet and bitter, which is evidenced by the change in the frequency of our swallowing in our fetal state. Thus, when we perceive a sweet taste, we have more swallowing movements of amniotic fluid than when we perceive something bitter.

This implies that our taste preferences are already being defined in the fetal state (Gestated Taste). The fetus is already able to distinguish between the taste of kale (unpleasant facial expression) and the taste of carrot (pleasant facial expression), and between the taste of aniseed or not[42,43] .

It is also capable of perceiving the textures (hard-soft, smooth-rugged, rough-soft, etc.) of the substances in dilution that reach the amniotic fluid, in order to get to know the different tastes of the different substances that our mother incorporates into her organism, since what the mother eats can also reach the amniotic fluid.[44] . Moreover, all ingestion is surrounded by an emotional, affective (feelings) and reasoning state. "My emotions, feelings and reasoning as a mother, influence the perception of taste of the child I am carrying", this influence is carried out by two ways, the first is by the degree of appetite that the mother has for a certain type of food; if she frequently eats a certain type of food, very frequently the embryo/fetus will receive, via the umbilical cord, the products of the digestion of that type of food, therefore the future baby will already have an apprenticeship for certain foods; The second way, the most important, is the transmission, from the mother to the fetus, of the positive or negative emotions produced by a certain food intake, this happens through the effect of the neurotransmitters and hormones released by the mother, when she experiences the "pleasantness" or "unpleasantness" of what she eats, since the hormones of the sensation of (Dopamine, Serotonin, Oxytocin, Adrenalin) are different from those of the sensation of "unpleasantness" (Cortisol). Since these substances circulate in the bloodstream, they pass from the mother to the fetus, causing in the fetus the same effects that the mother has had: pleasure or discomfort. In this way, when he is born to his life as a baby, the perception of certain tastes will cause him attraction or repulsion depending on what the mother experienced while he was a fetus, in fact we should say: what he experienced during his fetal life.

But apart from what happens during gestation, once the fetus passes to the newborn stage, a new sensory dimension is built, it is a new form of transtaste. We are referring to the fact that the nerves of the senses, apart from having the function of managing the perception of the sense they control, have other functions. If we take the nerves that participate in the gustatory function such as the Facial Nerve, the Glossopharyngeal Nerve, the Vagus Nerve and the Trigeminal Nerve, we will see, for example, that the Vagus Nerve, which captures the taste of the pharynx region, also acts on the ear, the lungs, the aorta artery, the heart, the esophagus, the stomach, liver, pancreas, intestine and immunity[45] . What does this mean? It means that all these actions are linked to taste and vice versa (taste is linked to all other functions). This example confirms, first, that each of these nerves has other actions in addition to those of taste, and second, that these actions are influenced by taste and vice versa. Thus, for example, if instead of referring to the Vagus Nerve, we refer to the Facial Nerve, which also participates in taste, we must include, in addition to taste, the functions on the musculature of facial expression and on hearing (audition). Regarding the glossopharyngeal nerve, it has a general sensory function on the tonsils, pharynx, Eustachian tube (ear), middle ear, posterior third of the tongue, and carotid sinus (arterial and chemical pressure). There remains the trigeminal nerve, whose territory is very large. It is in charge of the touch (pressure, temperature, viscosity, humidity, pungency, etc.) of the anterior 2/3 of the tongue, it also has muscular and auditory actions, pain perception, parotid gland, masticatory muscles, musculature and sensitivity of the eyes, nose, forehead, jaw, teeth, facial skin, anterior area of the head and intracranial region (dura mater).

The link between the sense of taste and other bodily functions is thus clear.

Later, already in the extrauterine life, the attraction or rejection will be remodeled by cultural influences (family, friends, etc.) that will modify the degrees of appetite for certain types of foods.

Our sense of taste, which as we have already seen, is connected with smell, touch, with the other senses, with the rest of the body's organs, and now we add that it is linked, especially with your microbiome.

The human body contains, for a 70 kg person, $(3.72+ 0.8)x10^{13}$ cells in his body, which in round numbers is about 40 billion/70kg = 4 billion /7 kg = 4000 million/7g = 571 billion/gr. of cells of which between 86 billion and 100 billion are found in the brain. Most of these cells are renewed almost every 10 years.[46,47,48,49] . It is assumed that there are about ten bacteria for every cell, and about ten viruses for every bacterium in our body. We can have a comparison to see the proportions, in this case, between the microbial endowment of a person and the amount of cells possessed in general, compared to the number of neurons (Fig. 29).

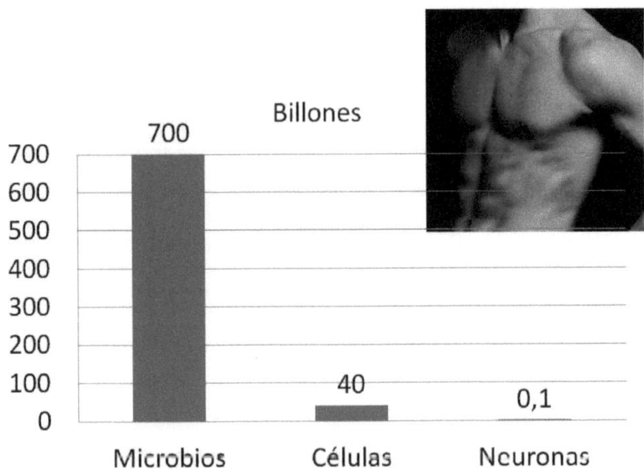

Fig. 29. Our body contains about 700 trillion microbes, while the number of body cells, on average, is about 40 trillion cells, which at the brain level would correspond to about 100 billion neurons.

Our microbial endowment, our global microbiome contains, apart from the external microbiome located in the skin, the internal microbiome located in the digestive system. The genetics that we possess together with our habits (food and non-food) that we have, condition the conditions of our microbiome. The mistreatment or the good treatment that we have on it, will have repercussions on the general state of the body and the person. The microbial flora of our digestive system, which goes from the oro-pharynx to the anal region, is in charge of transforming what we ingest into usable products for the rest of the organism, at the same time that they supply us with vitamins, enzymes, hormones, etc., and they keep the toxins. and they keep the toxins. When we mistreat the digestive microbiome, by means of incorrect diets and states of stress, the set of microbes that thanked us for the good treatment we had with them, stops collaborating in the digestion (elaboration of nutrients), stops providing us with vitamins, enzymes, hormones, etc., stops absorbing toxins and what is worse, floods our body with the toxins that they produce.

This situation ends up having repercussions on the rest of the body, and therefore on the senses, altering, among them, the sense of taste. This type of alteration of our microbiome, of our bacterial flora, is called Intestinal Dysbacteriosis.

Human beings can live thanks to their coexistence with the microbial world. The balance maintained between the two allows the proper functioning of both.

There are, however, circumstance(s) that can alter the taste, for different reasons, which will act on the microbiome of the person. It is the work world (working with certain chemical substances), the clinical history of the person (the set of diseases he/she has suffered or suffers from) and especially, in this last section, it should be taken into account the medications he/she is taking, since they are the most common cause of taste alterations (dysgeusias), in the latter case its action is directly chemical on the taste receptors and sensors.

It remains for us to refer to toxic habits, such as alcohol intake, tobacco and other types of drugs, as elements that influence the perception of taste.

8-From Memory to Disgust (from oral to moral)

Everything that has been learned throughout life leaves a sediment, a dregs that we can call memory. Memory encompasses all the dimensions of the human being that are based on events of the stimulus-response type. Some of these types of events give rise to sensory experiences that, in turn, provoke a form of response that we call emotions, which are the cause of the emergence of feelings that will be the engine of reasoning.

From reasoning we see that the mind generates thoughts, which become ideas, which give rise to beliefs that in turn will generate criteria, from which will arise values that will be the reference points of the person on which his attitudes will be established, from which his habits (actions) will be configured.

This long chain of events is stored in "memory" format, which is the basis for memories and project management.

There are different types of memory[50,51,52] that we will only list (Fig. 30). This complexity of different types of memory are the pillars that clothe our memories and allow us to make projects based on our experience.

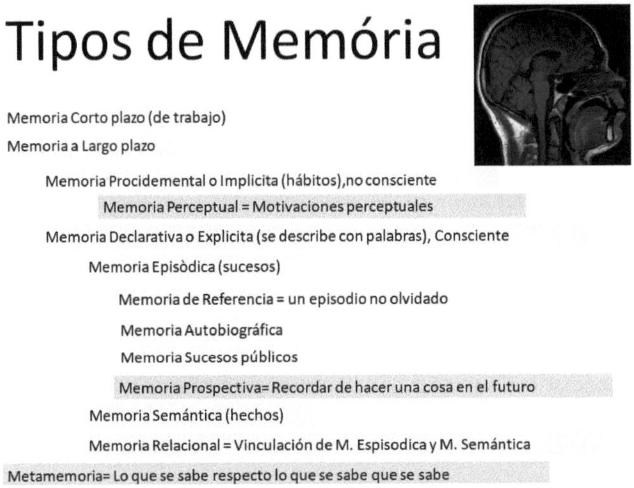

Tipos de Memória

Memoria Corto plazo (de trabajo)

Memoria a Largo plazo

Memoria Procidemental o Implicita (hábitos),no consciente

Memoria Perceptual = Motivaciones perceptuales

Memoria Declarativa o Explicita (se describe con palabras), Consciente

Memoria Episòdica (sucesos)

Memoria de Referencia = un episodio no olvidado

Memoria Autobiográfica

Memoria Sucesos públicos

Memoria Prospectiva= Recordar de hacer una cosa en el futuro

Memoria Semántica (hechos)

Memoria Relacional = Vinculación de M. Espisodica y M. Semántica

Metamemoria= Lo que se sabe respecto lo que se sabe que se sabe

Fig. 30 Different types of memory. In yellow, everything that depends on the hippocampus (most important area of memory) which is retrospective. In blue, it does not depend on the hippocampus.

Taste experiences are recorded in memory, together with all the other surrounding experiences, hence the appetite for a particular taste is sought or rejected according to the mnesic record (memory). As we can see, and we are repeating, taste is less and less the classical concept of perceiving basic sensations, and more the elements that surround it (Fig. 31). It is nothing more than taking up the concept that genetics does not exist alone, but depends on epigenetics. It is the genetic-epigenetic unit.

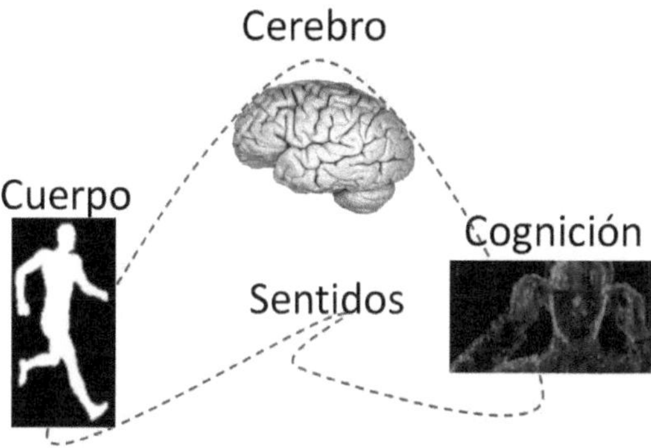

Fig. 31 Taste is influenced by what happens to the body, brain, senses and knowledge.

The rejection of a certain taste, due to the disgust that a food can produce in us, well, this type of response of repugnant character is located in the **anterior insula** of our brain. It has also been proven that the "disgust" brain centers are located in the same place as the place where the "moral criteria" are managed, the **anterior insula**. This same brain area is where alexithymia occurs, which consists of the difficulty in describing oneself through words, one's emotions and feelings (Fig. 32,33,34,35,36)[53,54] .

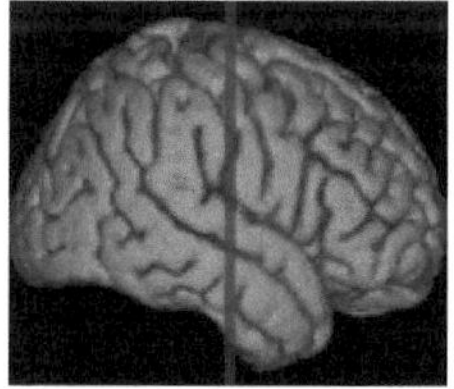

Fig. 32 Location of the insula is at the level of the vertical line in its lower third. The right side of the image is the anterior part of the brain, and the left side is the posterior part. This would be a person looking to the right.

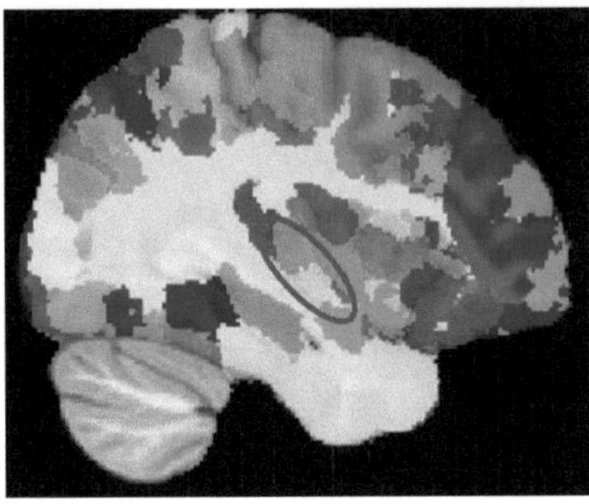

Fig. 33 Location of the insula (red circle) of a person looking to the right.

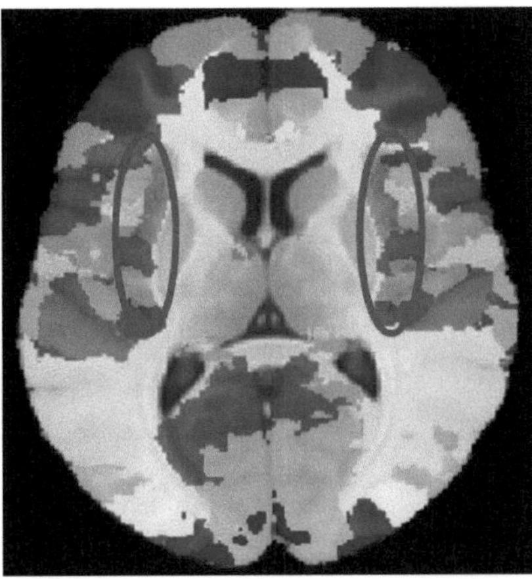

Fig. 34 Location of the two insulae (red circle) on the side D and I. The upper part corresponds to the frontal or anterior area of the head, and the lower part corresponds to the posterior area of the head.

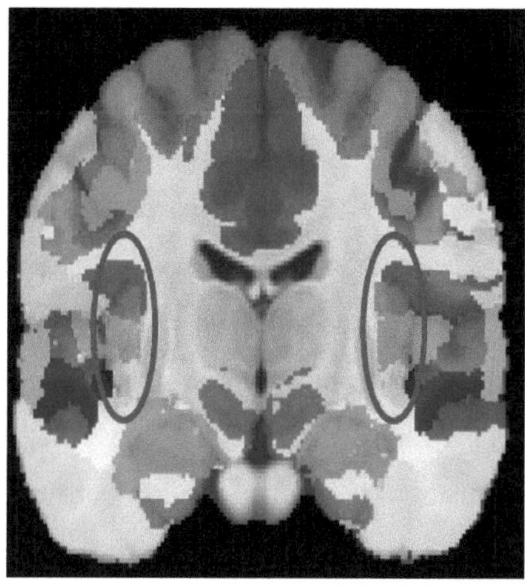

Fig. 35 Location of the Insula (red circle). The two insulae D and I, of a person who would be looking at us.

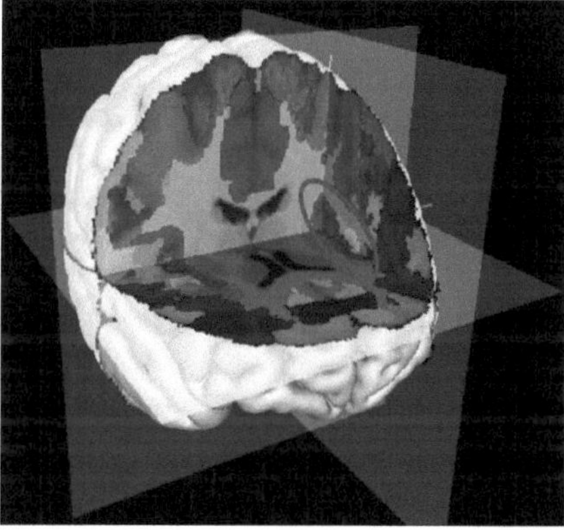

Fig. 36 Location of the insula (red circle) in a three-dimensional view of a person who would be looking towards us.

But not only taste, disgust, revulsion and alexithymia are managed in the Insula, but also social pain (evolved extension of physical pain) and morality are processed in the same area.

Our brain is able to distinguish between a computer and a person, and it does so in the insula, which is more active in front of a person than in front of an image of a person on a computer screen[55] . It is as if there is more empathy for a person than for his or her image. The insula processes the pleasantness or unpleasantness that one has before an Object, an Event or a Subject; as a result, there is a link with justice, more specifically with injustice[56] . The previous Insula shows aversion, injustice, disgust to bodily fluids (drinking one's own saliva), incest, or homosexuality in conservative people. Thus, we find that our brain shows our scientific, philosophical and political tendencies in the same area of taste. Taste is linked to both the physical and mental (moral and ethical) worlds.

9-From oral to moral

When we taste what we do is an ingestion of something. For ingestion to be correct there must be digestion and excretion. **Ingestion-Digestion-Excretion constitute a unit (IDE)**. (Fig. 37).

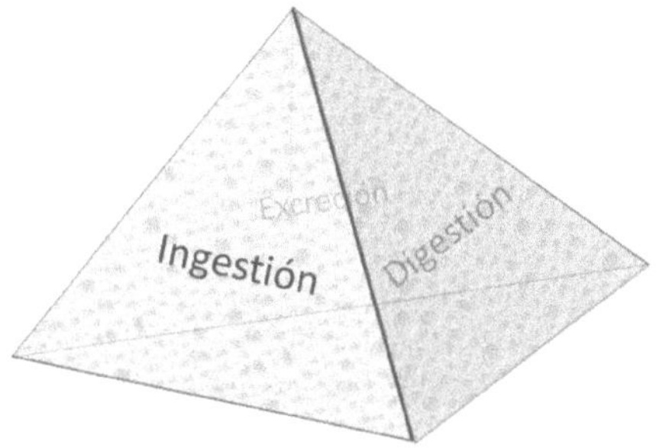

Fig. 37. IDE (Ingestion-Digestion-Excretion) Unit

Oral ingestion is not the only form of ingestion in our organism. We have air ingestion (respiratory), oral ingestion (solids and liquids), cutaneous ingestion (solids, liquids, gases, radiations), sensory ingestion (organoleptic), affective ingestion (feelings) and reasoning (ideas) (Fig.38,39 and 40). (Fig.38,39 and 40).

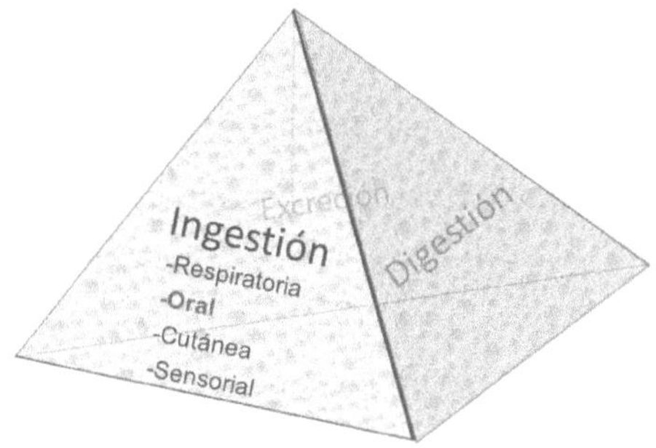

Fig. 38. IDE unit with all input paths

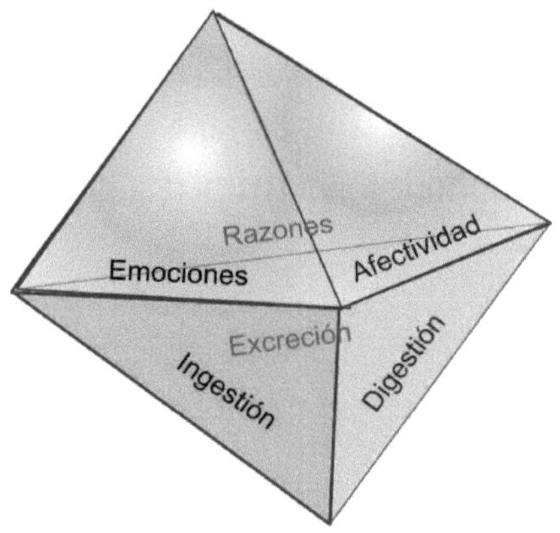

IDE unit linked to ingestions, digestions and excretions of emotions, affectivity and reasons.

All ingestion must be processed (digestion) and its waste eliminated (excretion), whether it is solid, liquid, gas, radiation, emotions, feelings (affective) or reasons. Our metabolism requires these steps, both at a material and cognitive level. What we ingest, in whatever format it is, is processed and cannot be accumulated, it must only remain in us in the form of its effects and influences, and the rest must be expelled. If what we ingest as liquids, solids and gases, we process and get rid of their residues, in order not to accumulate them, our emotions, feelings and reasons have to go through the same stages. If we cannot accumulate what is in material format, neither can we accumulate the non-material formats of our perceptions, whether they are in the form of emotions, feelings or reasons. For the simple reason that they do not fit in us. They can only, in part, be stored in the form of memory of what happened. The sense of taste suffers from such stages.

At this point, and going further, we can speak of "disgust" (Dis-taste, or alteration of taste). This concept allows us to refer both to a bad taste, from the point of view of taste, and to a way of acting, doing or carrying because of bad news. The leap here we see is qualitative, we speak of disgust at a cockroach, incest, defecation, etc., which activate the emotional response system to disgust, such as non-verbal expression, nausea and rejection[57] , which are managed in the same brain territory of taste that we call Insula.

If we leave behind the classical concepts that have governed the world of the senses, and enter into the new conception of Sensory Perception defined as the unit of **sensory-sensory-perceptual** units of our cognitive state that makes us conscious, we can observe that our sensory organs, among them taste, are in charge of collecting external stimuli and sending them to the sensory territories of the brain where they can be processed in the form of perception ("awareness of what is happening"), among them taste, are in charge of collecting external stimuli and sending them to the sensory territories of the brain where they can be processed in the form of perception ("awareness of what is happening"), which is why our senses must be seen as a part of the structure of consciousness. To want to separate the sensory organ from its sensory brain area and its link with perception is a very important mistake, since it has been demonstrated the reciprocal influence between the sensory organs, their own brain areas and the rest of the areas that convert this link into a consolidated perception. One way to understand this complex mechanism is to fragment our brain function (artificially) into **7 systems** that affect all the senses including taste, which are:

1-The Audio-Otico-Acoustic **(AOA),**

2-The Oculo-Ophthalmic-Visual **(OOV),**

3-Naso-Pupillo-Pupillary-Olfactory **(NPO)**

4-Oro-Faringo-Gusto-Sapido, where we find the taste **(OFGS)**.

To which we must add the following systems:

5-The Osteo-Tendinous-Tendinous-Musculo-Somatic **(OTMS),**

6-The Vascular-Hematic-Metabolic **(VHM),**

7-The Neuro-Psycho-Emotional **(NPE)**.

Therefore, the brain area that constructs taste and disgust and morality are linked to these 7 systems, whose degree of optimal state will condition any perception. Having said this, we can ask ourselves what is the use of all this, and the answer is that the classical vision that was obtained until now, and where more global aspects were not taken into account, such as these structures in systems, did not allow us to understand aspects that appeared accompanying certain responses, which are part of taste. Thus, what we understand by "taste in the mouth" is expanded not only by what happens in the mouth and throat, but also by what happens in the set of taste receptors scattered throughout the body and by the blocks we have mentioned.

Both will be activated by stimulating the sense of taste, which will start with the vision of what we are going to eat **(OOV)**, which will be deposited in the mouth **(OFGS)**, will reach the retronasal area **(NPO)**, to which the sound of what we eat **(AOA)** will be added, initiating chewing and swallowing **(OTMS)**, which will provide nutrients **(VHM)** and will end up affecting the nervous system **(NPE)** that in one way or another will have repercussions on the cerebral areas of taste, which, in a linked way, will modulate disgust, morality and justice.

If we place ourselves in the territory, no longer of taste but of tasting, understood as "tasting or tasting food or drink, generally with delight", we must take into account the effects of three patterns which are the unity Body-Mind-Spirit; "Body, understood as the structured state of a matter and its function, the Mind understood as the structured state of thought, and the Spirit, understood as a philosophical-religious structured state" (Fig.40). It may seem strange to speak in these terms with respect to something as "prosaic" as eating. Let us take up again that the concept of eating (ingestion) requires digestion and excretion, which is a useful dynamic for all human levels.

Opening up to this new level constitutes the last frame where the consciousness of oneself and of the environment is constructed, which allows an oriented state of the person with respect to the place, time and situation, and which in medicine is called **"sensorium"**. The sensorium is influenced by the Body-Mind-Spirit unit, which in turn is influenced by the perception of the sense of taste, by disgust, by morality and justice (Fig.41).

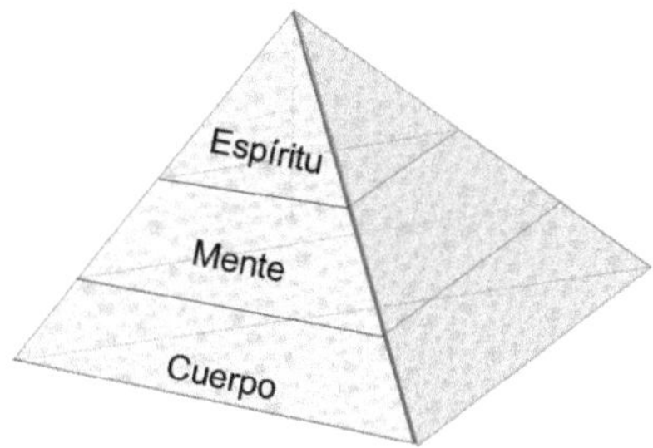

Fig. 40. It may seem strange, but it is impossible that the conditions of Body-Mind-Spirit do not influence the elaboration of taste and tasting.

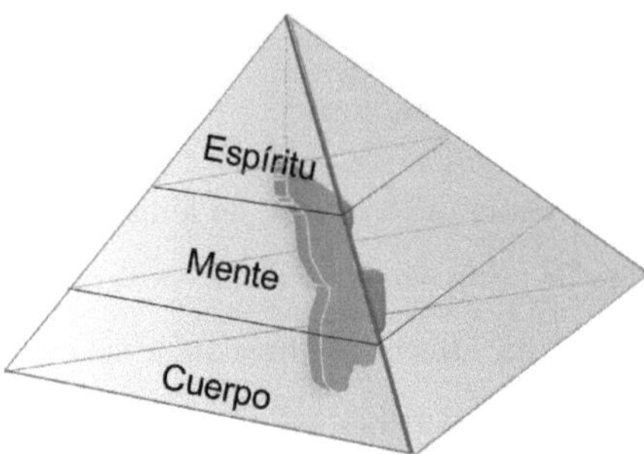

Fig. 41 The body-mind-spirit unity is part of the construction of taste and disgust. Conversely, what happens at the level of the body, mind and spirit of the person has repercussions on the perception of taste and disgust.

10-From Dysgeusia to Disgust/From Disgust to Dysgeusia

As a consequence of the knowledge we have about taste, to speak of alterations supposes, at least, to make reference to unilateral, bilateral, complete or partial lesions of the nerve fibers (cranial pairs) that are in charge of the perception of taste, all this would be part of the alteration of taste (dysgeusia), but as we have already been indicating we have to attend the extended vision to territories located beyond the mouth, throat and nose, which would configure the displeasure.

We are going to enter the territories of taste and disgust alteration, from different angles in order to have a more global vision. A concrete way to understand the multidisciplinary territory that encompasses taste in the mouth is that it is influenced by disgust (the displeasures we experience) and vice versa. The quality of satiation in the mouth determines the quality of satiation in the rest of the body (emotions, feelings and reasons), in other words, alterations of the "taste" type condition alterations of the "disgust" type and vice versa. Therefore, if we conceive Disgust as an emotional-feeling-reasoning state, we must bear in mind that taste plays in the same league.

The importance of this knowledge is not the number of specific discoveries that are provided, but the general conception that it brings of the global vision of our sensoriality applied to the sense of taste. This vision tells us about the interconnection of the 12 points (filters of perception) shown in figure 2, which shows us the filters of perception, and which we can now contemplate, with a different orientation in fig.42.

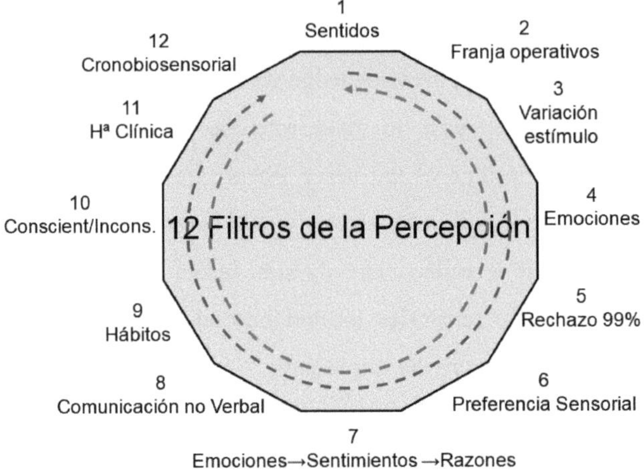

Fig. 42 Perceptual filters that act on taste

If we read the graph, according to the red dotted line (clockwise), we realize that it makes a lot of sense. From the senses we understand that each sense (nº1) will capture that for which it is prepared (nº2 = operative band) and that within this operative band, that sense will only be activated if there is a variation of the stimulus (nº3) and so on until reaching nº12; but if what we do is to read this graph in the opposite direction (green dotted line) (opposite direction to clockwise) a new interpretation appears to us since we would begin with nº 12 (Chronobiology) which would be telling us that depending on the moment of the day and the season of the year our Clinical History would modify filter nº11, which in turn would modify our states of consciousness (nº10)...and so on and so forth we would go backwards, seeing how each of these filters is modified and modifies the next one, and so following the green dotted line, we would arrive at the sense, at the senses that would also be modified. Now that we can see it in both directions (Fig. 42), we can realize that we are used to understanding physiology as a stimulus-response-unit to achieve an objective (from filter n°1 to 12), however, it is being suggested that what really happens is just the opposite: to achieve an objective we go in search of a stimulus-response (from filter n°12 to 1).

The first model would speak of the influence of the stimuli we receive and the consequences that arise in our organism and how we assimilate them, while the second model, which is currently proposed, consists in the fact that our objectives, our goals, seek the stimuli that activate the systems to achieve the desired goal[58] .

If we apply all this to the sense of taste, we can not only glimpse, but affirm that the sense of taste is linked to and depends on each of the processes we have been discussing. This vision is like saying, for example, with respect to salt and its salty taste, "My objective is to obtain some benefits for my body, for my health, for my perception, and for this I have to look for and find and use a certain stimulus, which in this case would be the taste of salt." Or what is the same: I conceive an objective and I look for the stimulus that helps me to achieve it, instead of saying: I look for a stimulus that gives me an objective , which would correspond to "I look for the taste of salt to achieve a stimulus to see what result it gives me".

11-An approach to diagnosis

We can start from the classic methodology based on a good clinical history, whose main part will be the anamnesis (interrogation), where we must know what questions to ask, to obtain the information that will guide us towards the etiology (cause) of the process.

We will begin with a general anamnesis: sex: age[59] , environment, work, habits, medical history (medical by devices and systems, surgical and therapeutic.). This should be followed by a specific anamnesis on the taste disorder (dysgeusia), which can be sudden, slow, permanent, cyclical - look for what the patient links it to (more often than we think the patient is right), discern whether it is a disorder of smell or taste (if it is the sense of smell that is altered, the patient will say that coffee is bitter, sweet or not depending on whether or not sugar has been added and hot, ice cream is cold and sweet, vinegar or lemon acid, aspirin is bitter, etc.), but if it is the taste that is altered, the patient will say that coffee is bitter, sweet or not depending on whether or not sugar has been added and hot, ice cream is cold and sweet, vinegar or lemon is acidic, aspirin is bitter, etc.).), but if it is the taste that is altered, you will not have any of these sensations, or only some of them, and you may even get a wound on the tongue by bites due to the anesthesia of the same without having the taste affected, due to the lesion of the nerve fibers of touch. We will then go on to investigate what happens in the 7 systems and the 3 levels. Discovering alterations in these areas will allow us to discover the type and degree of "disgust" that is hidden and that may be giving rise to a certain type of "disgust", which is influencing the perception of "classic" taste.

The second step is the physical examination of the oro-pharyngeal cavity, which will be followed by the exploration of the rest of the organs and otorhinolaryngological areas, in order to rule out distant processes such as otic (eardrum cord), nasal (trigeminal) or laryngeal (cranial nerve IX involvement) obstructions, etc. .

The third step consists of specific tests on taste and smell, not forgetting the latter since it is necessary to discern hidden pathologies on the sense of smell that can be interpreted as alterations of taste (usually happens when confusing taste with flavor). Taste, as we have already explained, is the perception of sapid characteristics such as sweetness, saltiness, acidity, etc., while flavor is the combination of taste + smell), so it will be necessary to perform olfactometry and gustometry. Gustometry has to explore the chemical-sensory function (sour, sweet, bitter, salty, umami tastes) by means of a chemogustometer. The somatosensory function (touch)[60] should also be explored by means of an electronic gustometer, the neurovegetative function by means of clinical anamnesis and explorations, and finally the neuropsychological function via Magnetic Resonance Imaging of taste.

The fourth step is in the complementary tests such as nasosinusal CT, brain MRI, sialography, general and sialoanalytical analysis and all those explorations that are required depending on the etiological suspicion (ear, gastroesophageal reflux, etc.).

The fifth step is to establish, from the examinations, a diagnosis of certainty or, failing that, of probability. Thanks to the exploration of taste, a diagnostic orientation can be given, without forgetting that dysgeusias are mostly discovered from olfactory disorders (only 13% of people who say they have lost their taste have really lost it, confusing the loss of aroma with the loss of taste).

With the data obtained from the examination we can group by systems the different etiologies that can be hereditary, congenital, neurological, psychiatric, otorhinolaryngological, lower respiratory tract, digestive, cardiovascular, nephro-urological, endocrine-sexual, neuromuscular, rheumatic, hematological, immunoallergic, dermatological, trauma, toxic (drugs, habits, work, environment), etc.[61,62] reaching up to 200 causes that alter the taste.

From the exploration of taste, which as we have seen is not exclusively gustometric, we can find the **"nosogeusia"** that deals with the pathology of taste in general, or the specific alteration called "**dysgeusia",** partial deficit: **"hypogeusia"**, and total deficit: **"ageusia"**. The excess: **"hypergeusia"**, the distortions: **"parageusia"**, those of bad taste: "**cacogeusia**", when one taste is interpreted by another (sweet taste in only salty foods): **"gustatory illusion**", when the taste is masked by predominance of another taste (for example, all, or most of the things like bitter): **"phantogeusia"** when there is fear of certain tastes by unpleasant experiences: "**geusiaphobia", and** when there is perception of a taste by the perception of a taste: **"phantogeusia", and when there is perception of a taste: "phantogeusia".** and when there is perception of a taste before a non-taste stimulus: **"gustatory hallucination"**.

Thus, thanks to the exploration of taste, a therapeutic approach and its follow-up can be offered. Instrumental techniques for the measurement of taste are based on parameters of intensity perception, perception of thresholds, identification and discrimination capacity, by means of different gustometers that can be of five main classes: (a) of subjective assessment whose range can go from being of chemical substances (sweet, salty, sour, bitter, bitter, umami) in dry form or in dilution or tactile-electronic (electrogustometers); b) of objective evaluation where we find Electroencephalographic Evoked Potentials of Taste (PEEGG), or Magnetoencephalography (MEG) or Gustatory Evoked Potentials (PEG),

Functional Magnetic Resonance Imaging (fMRI), Positron Emission Tomography (PET), etc., and c) objectification of subjective experiences[63] with which psychophysical scales and sensation explorations are applied by stimulus of the whole oral cavity, d) morphohistological explorations (videomicroscopic of the tongue), and e) by stimulations of neural territories, etc.

They can be used for studies in pathological processes that can be based on the type of stimulus (punctual or sustained stimuli) or on spatial aspects: a) of the whole oropharyngeal cavity, or only of specific geographic areas[64] (right, left, anterior, posterior, only the tongue, or only the palate, etc.), b) of specific types of papillae (fungiform, goblet, foliated, etc.), c) of specific areas of nerve terminals, e.g. the V pair for the general sensitivity of nerve terminals.), b) of specific types of papillae (fungiform, goblet, foliated), c) of only specific areas of nerve terminals, for example the V pair for the general sensitivity of the anterior 2/3 of the tongue (touch, textures, itching, pain, hardness, viscosity, etc.), or of the VII pair for the general sensitivity of the anterior 2/3 of the tongue (touch, textures, itching, pain, hardness, viscosity, etc.).), or the VII pair for taste sensitivity (sweet, salty and sour) in the anterior 2/3 of the tongue, and the IX pair for the study of the general sensitivity of the posterior 1/3 of the tongue and taste (bitter) and also of the pharyngo-larynx-esophageal area, where there are also taste terminals, the X pair for general sensitivity, d) study of the taste sensory pathways (from the tongue to the cortex). Studies can be done by age, sex and neuropsychological, neuropsychiatric, forensic studies. Each of these systems of taste exploration requires the adaptation of substances according to cultural habits (there are cultures with little habit to the use of salt, or cultures with a lot of habit to the ingestion of sweet, etc.).

The gustometric study does not end with the cranial pairs and the social habits, the situation of the neurovegetative pathways (sympathetic-parasympathetic) that are conveyed by the different cranial pairs must be analyzed, together with the linguo-pharyngo-laryngo-esophageal motricity (V, IX and XII pairs) where chewing and swallowing take shape, IX and XII pairs) where chewing and swallowing take shape, since taste is linked to these functions, this means that chewing-swallowing depend on general sensitivity, specific sensitivity and neurovegetative function; and conversely, general and specific sensitivity are dependent on motor and neurovegetative function.

Whichever method we use for taste exploration, we must bear in mind that any model of gustometer has particular limitations, depending on its design, and general limitations due to the scope of the territory it explores. Thus, the classic manual stimulation taste testers provide manageability, with little economic expense and accuracy of results, but with a tendency to lose global vision, while the latest generations of computerized taste testers provide global vision but are complex from the point of view of manageability and much more expensive, with a tendency to present local shortcomings. This being said, it is obvious that both can be complementary.

We can verify that the set of explorations that we have exposed, are part of the classic methodology of exploration, since the study of a) the **Ingestion-Digestion-Excretion that constitute the IDE unit,** b) the **sensory ingestion (organoleptic),** the **affective ingestion (Feelings)** and the **reasoning (ideas),** c) the **7 systems (pages 47 and 48)** and d) the **3 levels (Body, Mind and Spirit)** that would require extending the exposition that we have made both of the exploration and the diagnosis, remain outside of it.

As previously mentioned, all ingestion, digestion and excretion are linked. The greater the ingestion, the greater the digestion and the greater the excretion, the reverse is also true and in the opposite direction, a greater excretion means a greater ingestion, and therefore a greater digestion. Apart from the fact that not everything is ingestable, digestible and excretable, we have the problem of the loss of this correlation, such as eating a lot and digesting little, or eating little and digesting a lot, or eating a lot and digesting a lot but excreting very little, etc. To such an extent this is so, that any abuse of excess or lack of ingestion, digestion and excretion, at any of the different levels that have been exposed, alter the functioning of our senses, and as always, among them, the sense of taste. Taste is not independent of these events.

12-3OIKO^S Tasting menu

We will develop a global and final vision of the world of Taste, Tasting and Swallowing. These three functions are intertwined with what we call the 7C's (C^7). C^7 is the basic structure of the enjoyment of eating. C^7 refers to the Kitchen, the Cook, the Dining Room, the Meal, the Eater, the Clinic (of the kitchen, the cook, the dining room, the meal) and the Eating (Chewing, Salivating, Swallowing), and this C^7 . The world of taste is intimately linked to C^7 , the attention of taste implies the development of the seven territories exposed. Moreover, Taste, Tasting and Swallowing can no longer go on their own, they must be in harmony with the environment.

Let's imagine that we are walking down the street, looking for a restaurant to satisfy our hunger, we see one that attracts us by name: Restaurant "3OIKO^S ", we had never seen it before, it seems new and our curiosity to know more about it, leads us to enter to find out and satisfy our dining experience. We ask if we can eat, they tell us yes and offer us a table, to which we go and sit down. Soon after, he brings us the menu where we find the menu that says:

"Bios Oikologicós starters".

Second: "Prosopon Oikoumené style".

"Oikonomikós Glykýs desserts".

It takes almost no time to bring us the starter of Bios Oikologicós, and as we do not know what the hell is each of the dishes on the menu, which by discretion, at first, we have not enjoyed asking what they were made of, and tucking us with the trick of letting us be surprised, we ask him to explain them to us. He tells us that the name of the starter comes from the Greek βίος (Bios) which means "life" and from the also Greek word οἶκος (Oikos) which means "house", place where one lives and from which arises the Greek word οἰκολογία (oikologia) that we know as **"Ecology"**, It is a dish that tells us about life at the ecological level. The second dish the Oikoumené style Prosopon, whose name also comes from the Greek πρόσωπον (Prosopon) which means "person", and from the Greek word οἰκουμένη (Oikouménē) which also contains the prefix "oiko "and means "inhabited land" and that we know with the word "Ecumenical" remaining the idea of **"Ecumenical Person"**. In this case the dish refers to the earth inhabited by the human being. The last dish, the dessert named Oikonomikós Glykós, comes from the same language as the previous ones, it is composed of oîkos "house" and νέμειν (némein) which means 'distribute', 'manage' and from which arises οἰκονομία (Oikonomia) which we know as **"Economy",** while γλυκός (Glykós) means "sweet"**.** It is a dessert that wants to remind us that the economy, the administration does not have to be something rough and unpleasant, but rather kind.

Thus it turns out that we have ingested the components of a menu elaborated from the vision of the Ecological, the Ecumenical and the Economic. We soon realize that this argumentative articulation must be applied to the knowledge of taste, of which we have written.

Nowadays nothing is spared, not even our sensory functions from the Ecological (of the degraded environment), Ecumenical (of dehumanized human beings) and Economic (of scarcity) effects. Our sensoriality, our senses, and among them taste, are being affected by the lack of respect for the environment, the lack of human respect, and the lack of respect for basic and raw materials for all. Let's see an example in which we will focus briefly on the circumstance of one of the alterations that does not allow the person who suffers it, to be able to enjoy, not the menu that we have exposed, but any menu, for being one of the most important alterations that participate in the disorders of the ingestion, it is the Dysphagia.

On the one hand, we know that at least 200 diseases have been diagnosed with taste alterations, and on the other hand, we have an example of a disease known as "dysphagia", which is characterized by the alteration of swallowing dynamics and which often accompanies other causes of taste alterations.

Dysphagia" should be understood as an alteration in the ability to swallow that involves complications such as coughing, choking, aspiration, pulmonary diseases, malnutrition, cognitive impairment and quality of life. It is estimated that 1 in 17 people (5.8%) of the world's population suffer or will suffer some degree of dysphagia during their lifetime[65] , this means, for the current population of our planet of about 8,181,649,380 people (May 2024), that there are about 474,535,664 people with dysphagia. There are multiple studies in each country that show the rate of affectation, for example in the USA, there are according to different reports between 2% and 20% of the population with dysphagic affectation[66] . Therefore, this is a serious alteration that participates hindering the appreciation of taste, tasting, flavor and swallowing. It is worth considering, according to the set of parameters exposed, what kind of actions can be implemented for the care of people suffering from this pathology.

We know that the main tool for their attention, within the C^7 , is the set of physical characteristics of the food to be ingested, and specifically we also know that the most important of the characteristics is the degree of viscosity,[67] that the food to be ingested must present, depending on the degree of dysphagia of the person and the general state of the same, without forgetting that in the C^7 we find the Kitchen, the Cook, the Dining Room, the **Food**, the Eater, the Clinic (of the kitchen, of the cook, of the dining room, of the food) and the **Eating** (Chewing, salivating, swallowing).

I refer to this pathology as an example-claim of everything that should be included in the study of taste. Dysphagia is a clear example of a territory where each and every one of the exposed elements of current knowledge about the world of taste can be applied.

Educating our senses is a crucial task, since it means that it must be done in an Ecological, Ecumenical and Economic way. Let us put a final point with a general vision of taste, which is altered when we do not allude to $3OIKO^S$, when this happens, when we do not act in $3OIKO^S$, new alterations appear in the human being, which evidently leave the taste altered, are an example of this:

-Ecoanxiety, understood as the chronic fear of suffering an environmental cataclysm. The experience of the destruction of the environment is the cause of my anxiety levels.

The "Solastalgia"[68] , a term coined by Glenn Albrecht who defined it as the set of psychological disorders that occur in a native population, after destructive changes in their territory either as a result of human activities or climate. He also coined the term "Somaterratica" understood as the study of the pathological aspects, such as skin problems, due to the fact of being disconnected from nature. He also coined the term "Symbiocene" understood as a positive and symbiotic relationship between humans and nature.

-Uppgivenhetssyndrom[69] . It is a syndrome based on a claudication, a resignation, which appears in refugee children and adolescents in Sweden. It arises when they learn that their families will be deported to their countries. And finally, Hikikomori syndrome, which literally means "to withdraw, to be secluded", is a mental disorder that leads to social isolation of the patient. It is usually associated with psychosis, anxiety, depression[70] .

In this type of alterations, what is evident is the rupture of the principles of 3OIKO[S] with the total sensory alteration. Our sense of taste is part of multiple territories and as such must be attended to. The globality of the sense of taste and its other functions can only be sustained in the 3OIKOS dimension[S] .

Bibliography

1 Heckmann JG, Heckmann SM, Lang CJG, et al.Hummel T. Neurological Aspects of Taste Disorders. JAMA Neurologyc.2003 *Arch Neurol.* 2003;60(5):667-671. doi:10.1001/archneur.60.5.667.

2 Isaacson W. Einstein: His life and his universe (Biographies and Memoirs). Edt. Debate 2020

3 Köster, E P, Dgel J, Piper D. "Proactive and Retroactive Interferences in implicit Odor Memory". *Chemical Senses.* 2002.Vol. 27 Iss.3; pg 191.

4 Bensafi M, Rouby C, Farget V, Bertrand B, et al." Autonomic Nervous System Responses to Odours: the Role of Pleasantness and Arousal" *Chemical Senses. Oxford*: Oct 2002. Vol. 27, Iss. 8; pg. 703

5 Owen A M, Coleman MR, Boly M. et al. "Detecting Awareness in the Vegetative State". Science. Vol 313, 8 Sept 2006.

6 Díez Noguera A. "Biological rhythms in living beings". Chrono biology, pharmacology, pathology, Editors: Tamargo J., Barberà JM. Ed. Mayo. 2005, p. 1-20

7 Miller, Inglis J. Jr. and Linda M. Bartoshuk. Taste bud distribution and spatial relationships, pp. 205-234. Smell and Test in Health and Disease. Ed. by T.V. Getchell et al. Raven Press. New York. 1991.

8 Briand L and Salles C. Taste perception and integration. Chapter - December 2016 DOI: 10.1016/B978-0-08-100295-7.00004-9

9 Wilson-Pauwels L, Akesson EJ, Stewart PA. Spacey SD. Cranial nerves in health and disease. Secd Edt. Edt. BC Decker Inc. 2002.

10 Delwiche JF, Lera MF and Breslin A.S. Selective Removal of a Target Stimulus Localized by Taste in Humans. Chem. Senses 25:181-187, 2000.

11 Prof. Doron Lancet's research is supported by the Jeans-Jacques Brunschwig Fund for the Molecular Genetics of Cancer; Crown Human Genome Center; Avraham and Judy Goldwasser Fund; and Alfried Krupp

von Bohlen und Halbach Foundation. Prof. Lancet is the incumbent of the Ralph and Lois Silver Professorial Chair in Human Genomics. Weizmann Institute (2003, August 12). Weizmann Institute Scientists Report Why Taste And Smell Differ Among Individuals. SCIENCEDAILY. Retrieved July 26, 2010, from http://www.sciencedaily.com /releases/2003/08/030812073446.htm.2010

12 Kandel ER, Schwatz JH and Jessell TM. Smell and taste: the chemical senses. Principles of Neuroscience. Fourth Edt. Mcgraw-Hill, Interamericana: 624-647. 2001.

13 Purves D, Augustine GJ, Fitzpatrick D, et al. Chemical senses; 287-314. Invitation to Neuroscience. Edt. Médica Panamericana. 2004

14 Bartosshuk Linda M. Comparing sensory Experiencies Across Individuals: Recent Psychophysical Advances Illuminate Genetic Variation in taste Perception. Chem. Senses 25: 447-460, 2000.

15 Taste perception and integration. Loic Briand and Christian Salles. Chapter - December 2016 DOI: 10.1016/B978-0-08-100295-7.00004-9

16 Laugerette, F; Passilly-Degrace, P; Patris, B; Niot, I; Febbraio, M; Montmayeur, J. P.; Besnard, P (2005). "Involvement of CD36 in orosensory detection of dietary lipids, spontaneous fat preference and digestive secretions". *Journal of Clinical Investigation* **115** (11): 3177-84. PMC 1265871. PMID 16276419. doi:10.1172/JCI25299.

17 Dipatrizio, N. V. (2014). "Is fat taste ready for primetime?". *Physiology & Behavior*. 136C: 145-154. PMC 4162865. PMID 24631296. doi:10.1016/j.physbeh.2014.03.002.

18 Wei ET, Seid DA (1983). "AG-3-5: a chemical producing sensations of cold". J. Pharm. Pharmacol. **35** (2): 110-2

19 Romera E,,Perena MJ,,Perena MF,,and Rodrigo MD. Neurophysiology of pain. R e v. Soc. Esp. Pain 7: Suppl. II, 11-17, 2000.

20 Sacre-Hazouri JA and Sacre L. Chronic cough. Cough reflex hypersensitivity syndrome. Rev Allerg Mex;66(2):217-231. 2019.

21 https://www.researchgate.net/publication/51535853

Moran MM, Allen McAlexander M, Bíró T and Szallasi A. Transient receptor potential channels as therapeutic Nature Reviews Drug Discovery 601-620 August 2011 DOI: 10.1038/nrd3456

22 Ana Gabriela Medina Torres (Algology, INCMNSZ). Bibliographic Review: Nociceptive TRP channels in multiple pain pathologies.

http://www.dolorypaliativos.org/dolorypaliativos/art386.asp

23 Brauchi S, Orta G, Mascayano C, Salazar M, Raddatz N, Urbina H, Rosenmann E, Gonzalez-Nilo F, and Latorre M*§ PNAS vol. 104 no. 24. 10246-10251. June 12, 2007.

24 Galán Martínez C, Souto Cárdenas R D, Valdés García S, Minaberriet Conceirol E. Transient Potential Receptor ion channels and their leading role in analgesic therapy. Cuban Journal of Biomedical Research. 2015; 34(3):278-288

25 https://www.bionity.com/es/noticias/1172999/premio-nobel-de-fisiologia-o-medicina-2021-concedido-a-los-cientificos-estadounidenses-david-julius-y-ardem-patapoutian.html

26 Lee S-J, Depoortere I and Hatt H.Therapeutic potential of ectopic olfactory and taste receptors. NATURE Reviews | DRug Discovery Reviews. volume 18 | FEBRUARY 2019 | 125. 2019

27 Mosingera B, Reddinga KM, Rockwell Parkera M, Yevshayevab V, Yeea KK, Dyominaa K, Lia Y, and Margolskeea RF. Genetic loss or pharmacological blockade of testes-expressed taste genes causes male sterility. PNAS | July 23, 2013 | vol. 110 | no. 30 | 12319-12324. 2013

28 Shaw L, Mansfield C, Colquitt L, Lin C, Ferreira J, Emmetsberger J, Reed DR. Personalized expression of bitter 'taste' receptors in human skin PLOS ONE |https://doi.org/10.1371/journal.pone.0205322 October 17, 2018.

29 Lee RJ, Xiong G, Kofonow JM, et al. T2R38 taste receptor polymorphisms underlie susceptibility to upper respiratory infection. The Journal of Clinical Investigation http://www.jci.org Volume 122 Number 11 November 2012

30 Lee J, Kofonow JM, Rosen PL et al. Bitter and sweet taste receptors regulate human upper respiratory innate immunity. The Journal of Clinical Investigation http://www.jci.org Volume 124 Number 3 March 2014.

31 Maßberg D and Hatt H. HUMAN OLFACTORY RECEPTORS: NOVEL CELLULAR FUNCTIONS OUTSIDE OF THE NOSE. *Physiol Rev* 98: 1739-1763, 2018.

32 https://invdes.com.mx/wp-content/uploads/2017/11/19-11-17-receptores-gustativos.jpg

https://mail.google.com/mail/u/0/?ogbl#inbox?projector=1

33 Shahid R.A. Erdmann A. et al. Neuroepithelial circuit formed by innervation of sensory enteroendocrine cells. J Clin Invest. 2015;125(2):782-786. doi:10.1172/JCI78361.

34 Buchanan KL, Rupprecht LE, Kaelberer MM et al The preference for sugar over sweetener depends on a gut sensor cell. Nature Neuroscience | VOL 25 | February 2022 | 191-200 | www.nature.com/natureneuroscience

35 Jérémy Chéret J, Bertolini M, Ponce L, Lehmann J, Tsai T, Alam M, Hatt H & Paus R.Olfactory receptor OR2AT4 regulates human hair. Growth. NATURE COMMUNICATIONS | DOI: 10.1038/s41467-018-05973-0

36 Manteniotis W, Wojcik S, Brauhoff P, Möllmann M, Petersen L, Göthert JR, Schmiegel W, Dührsen U, Gisselmann G and Hatt H.. Functional characterization of the ectopically expressed olfactory receptor 2AT4 in human myelogenous leukemia. Cell Death Discovery (2016) 2, 15070; doi:10.1038/cddiscovery.2015.70. © 2016 Cell Death Differentiation Association

37 MartineMartinez A , Ortega O, Viñas P et al. COVID-19 is associated with oropharyngeal dysphagia and malnutrition in hospitalized patients during the spring 2020 wave of the pandemic. https://doi.org/10.1016/j.clnu.2021.06.010.

38 Ebihara T, Ebihara S, Watando A, Okazaki T, Asada M, Ohrui T, Yamaya M &. Arai H. Effects of menthol on the triggering of the swallowing reflex in elderly patients with dysphagia. Br J Clin Pharmacol. 62:3 369-371.2006.

39https://patentimages.storage.googleapis.com/39/f9/63/054e4ee79f4852/EP3119385B2.pdf

40https://www.meiji.ac.jp/cip/english/news/2020/enjsp3000000f32u.html

41 https://www.dailymail.co.uk/sciencetech/article-11644933/Japanese-scientists-develop-electric-spoon-zaps-tongue-enhance-foods-salty-taste.html

42 Beyza Ustun1 , Nadja Reissland1 , Judith Covey1, Benoist Schaal2, and Jacqueline Blissett3 Flavor Sensing in Utero and Emerging Discriminative Behaviors in the Human Fetus. Psychological Science *XX(X)*1-12. 2022

43Schaal B, Marlier L, and Soussignan R. Human Foetuses Learn Odours from their Pregnant Mother's Diet. Chem. Senses 25: 729-737, 2000.

44 de Haro Licer J. Prenatal sensory-perception. Prenatal pedagogy of sensory perception. Edt. Autografía.2023.

45 https://www.nature.com/articles/d41586-024-01259-2?utm_source=Live+Audience&utm_campaign=52cfde5305-nature-briefing-daily-20240502&utm_medium=email&utm_term=0_b27a691814-52cfde5305-50955552

46 Azevedo F.A. C, Carvalho LR B, Grinberg L T, Farfel J M, Ferretti R E L, Leite R E P, Jacob Filho W, Lent R, Herculano-Houzel S. Equal numbers of neuronal and nonneuronal cells make the human brain an isometrically scaled-up primate brain. J Comp Neurol. 2009 Apr 10;513(5):532-41. doi: 10.1002/cne.21974.

47 Herculano-Houzel S .The human brain in numbers: a linearly scaled-up primate brain. Neurosci, 09 November 2009. Sec. Cognitive Neuroscience Volume 3 - 2009 | https://doi.org/10.3389/neuro.09.031.2009

48 Spalding KL Bhardwaj RD , Buchholz BA, Druid H. Frisén J, Retrospective Birth Dating of Cells in Humans..Vol 122, no. 1 , July 15, 2005, Pages 133-143.

49 E. Bianconi et al.. An estimation of the number of cells in the human body. Ann Hum Biol, Early Online: 1-11. 2013.+ DOI: 10.3109/03014460.2013.807878.

50 Eichenbaum H. Cognitive neuroscience of memory. Ariel 2003

51 Kandel ER. In search of memory. Birth of a new science of the mind. Katz Conocimiento.2007.

52 Johnson M. H. Developmental Cognitive Neuroscience. Blackwell Publishing. 2nd Edition. 2004.

53 Sophia K, Goerlich-Dobre, Lamm C, Prip J, Habel U, Votinov M.The left amygdala: A shared substrate of alexithymia and empathy.NeuroImage Jour. 122, pg. 22-32. 2015

54https://atlases.ebrains.eu/viewer/#/a:juelich:iav:atlas:v1.0.0:1/t:minds:core:referencespace:v1.0.0:dafcffc5-4826-4bf1-8ff6-46b8a31ff8e2/p:minds:core:parcellationatlas:v1.0.0:94c1125b-b87e-45e4-901c-00daee7f2579-300/@:0.0.0.-W000.._Uo56.2-MuCL._qr4O.2_FOAw..7Z1Y..29XHG.wSz4~.10gBm..5_zF

55 Takahashi H, Izuma K, Matsumoto M, Matsumoto K, Omori T. The Anterior Insula Tracks Behavioral Entropy during an Interpersonal Competitive Game. - PLoS ONE (2015).

56 Hsu M, Anen C and Quartz SR. The Right and the Good: Distributive Justice and Neural Encoding of Equity and Efficiency. VOL 320 SCIENCE. 23 MAY 2008. American Association for the Advancement of Sciencehttps://doi.org/10.1126/science.115365.

57 Rozin Paul, Haid Jonathan, Fincher Katrina. From Oral to Moral. Science vol. 323, 27 , pp. 1189-90Feb.2009.

58 Peña Casanova J and Sigg J. Towards an advanced Functional brain model (beyond Luria). Theory and interpretation. Normality. Neuropsychological semiology and pathology. Integrated neuropsychological screening program. Barcelona-2 test. Test-Barcelona. Services S.L.2019.

59 Cees de Graaf, Wija van Staveren and Jan Burema. Psychophysical and Psychohedonic Functions of Four Common Food Flavours in Elderly Subjects. Chemical Senses, 21: 293-304, 1996.

60 Bartosshuk, Linda M., Caseria, Donna, Catalanotto, Frank et al. Do taste-trigeminal interactions play a role in oral pain? Annual Meeting of Association for Chemoreception Sciences (AchemS XVIII). Chemical Sense... Volume 21, number 5, October Pag.578. 1996

61 Ackerman, Bruce H and Kasbekar, Nishaminy. Disturbances of Taste and Smell Induced by Drugs. Reviews of Therapeutics. Pharmacotherapy, 17 (3): 482-496. 1997

62 Pribitkin E, Rosenthal MD, Cowart B J. Prevalence and causes of severe taste loss in a chemosensory clinic population The Annals of

Otology, Rhinology & Laryngology. St. Louis. Vol. 112, Iss. 11; pg. 971: Nov 2003

63 Snyder DJ, Prescott J, Bartoshuk LM. Modern Psychophysics and the Assessment of Human Oral Sensation. Taste and Smell an Update. Advances in Oto-Rhino-Laryngology. Thomas Hummel, Antje Welge-Lüssen. Edt. Karger. Vol. 63. 2006.

64 Marion E. F, Hettingen E.P., Barry MA, et al. Contemporary Measurement of Human Gustatory Function. Doty RL. Handbook of Olfaction and Gustation. Second Edt. Marcel Dekker. 2003

65 Dysphagia Global guidelines and cascades. Gastroenterol. latinoam 2018; Vol 29, No. 4: 178-192.

66 Adkins C, Takakura W, Spiegel BMR, et al. Prevalence and Characteristics of Dysphagia Based on a Population-Based Survey. Clin Gastroenterol Hepatol. 2020 August ; 18(9): 1970-1979.e2. doi:10.1016/j.cgh.2019.10.029.

67 García González ML, García Raurich J, Raventós Santamaria M, Alba Mora M. Viscosity in the diet of patients diagnosed with oropharyngeal dysphagia. Acta Bioquím Clín Latinoam 2016; 50 (1): 45-60.

68 http://theobjective.com/further/el-sindrome-de-la-resignacion-una-extrana-enfermedad-que-se-ha-dado-a-conocer-en-el-world-press-photo/

69 Sallin K, LagercrantzH, Evers K, et al. . Resignation Syndrome: Catatonia? Culture-Bound? Front Behav Neurosci. 2016; 10: 7.doi: 10.3389/fnbeh.2016.00007 http://theobjective.com/further/el-sindrome-de-la-resignacion-una-extrana-enfermedad-que-se-ha-dado-a-conocer-en-el-world-press-photo/ .

70 Malagón-Amor A, Córcoles-Martínez D, Martín-López L M, Pérez-Solà V. *Hikikomori* in Spain: A descriptive study. *Int J Soc Psychiatry, 0020764014553003, first published on October 9, 2014.*

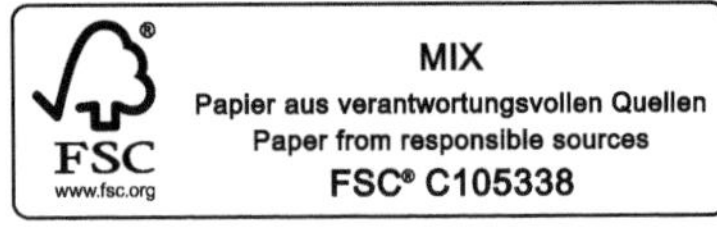

Printed by Books on Demand GmbH, Norderstedt / Germany